Frontiers of Primary Care

Series Editor: Mack Lipkin, Jr.

Frontiers of Primary Care

Series Editor: Mack Lipkin, Jr.

Henrietta N. Barnes Mark D. Aronson
Thomas L. Delbanco Editors

Alcoholism

A Guide for the Primary Care Physician

Foreword by Julius B. Richmond

With Contributions by A. Abrams, M.D. Aronson, H.N. Barnes, R.D. Bayog, M. Bean-Bayog, J. Bigby, B. Bush, M.G. Cyr, J. Daley, T.L. Delbanco, J. Ende, A.W. Fox, P.A. Friedman, M.E. Griner, P.F. Griner, M. Grodin, N.J. Guzman, A. Halliday, J.T. Harrington, K. Hesse, R.A. Hingson, A. Meyers, A.W. Moulton, S.F. O'Neill, J. Savitsky, W.A. Spickard, Jr., D.C. Walsh

Springer-Verlag
New York Berlin Heidelberg
London Paris Tokyo

Henrietta N. Barnes, M.D.
Instructor in Medicine,
Harvard Medical School,
Massachusetts General Hospital,
Chelsea Memorial Health Center,
Chelsea, MA 02150, USA

Mark D. Aronson, M.D.
Associate Professor of Medicine,
Harvard Medical School,
Beth Israel Hospital,
Boston, MA 02215, USA

Thomas L. Delbanco, M.D.
Associate Professor of Medicine,
Harvard Medical School,
Beth Israel Hospital,
Boston, MA 02215, USA

Series Editor
Mack Lipkin, Jr., M.D.
Director, Primary Care;
Associate Professor of Medicine,
New York University Medical
Center, School of Medicine,
New York, NY 10016, USA

With four Figures

Library of Congress Cataloging-in-Publication Data
Alcoholism : a guide for the primary care physician.
(Frontiers of primary care)
Includes index.
1. Alcoholism. 2. Family medicine. I. Barnes, Henrietta N. II. Aronson, Mark D. III. Delbanco, Thomas. IV. Abrams, A. (Alan), 1951– . V. Series.
[DNLM: 1. Alcoholism. WM 274 A35419]
RC565.A44518 1987 616.86'1 87-20652

Software reprint of the Hardcover 1st edition 1987

Typeset by Publishers Service, Bozeman, Montana.

ISBN-13: 978-1-4612-9155-8 e-ISBN-13: 978-1-4612-4786-9
DOI: 10.1007/978-1-4612-4786-9

9 8 7 6 5 4 3 2 1

To Our Families
David, Jacob, and Rebecca
Jean, Adam, Raney, Alexander, and Benjamin
Jill, Steve, Suzanne, and Jennifer

Series Preface

Primary care is the new frontier in medicine. Every nation worldwide has recognized the necessity to deliver personal and primary care to its people. This includes first contact care; care based in a positive and caring personal relationship; care by a single person for the majority of the patient's problems; coordination of all care by the patient's personal provider, advocacy for the patient; the provision of preventive and psychosocial care as well as care for episodes of acute and chronic illness. These facets of care work most effectively when embedded in a coherent integrated approach.

The support for primary care derives from several significant trends. First, technologically based care costs have rocketed beyond reason or availability. This has occurred in the face of exploding populations and diminishing real resources in many parts of the world, even in many parts of the wealthier nations. Simultaneously, the primary care disciplines—general internal medicine and pediatrics and family medicine—have matured significantly. They have become viable alternatives to the specialty approach to care with its potential dehumanization, coordination problems, and increased cost. The primary care disciplines have begun to create new sets of intellectual tools and new educational approaches to support their new paradigm of biopsychosocial care. These new tools include clinical epidemiology which examines the efficacy, effectiveness and efficiency of everyday, real world care; clinical decision making which is beginning to find ways to improve the rational basis for common clinical choice; the medical interview which is now coming under critical study as the major medium of care; problem based learning and community oriented medical education which enable efficient learning of the greatest relevance and with increased satisfaction for learner and teacher; and the philosophic and empiric study of ethical aspects of care.

A number of major questions have emerged in the new disciplines. Who is to do primary care? What do they need to know? How can the needed content, skills, and attitudes be best taught? Who is to teach these new practitioners and what skills do they need? The persons interested in these sorts of questions include practitioners, teachers, and researchers in primary medicine.

The Frontiers of Primary Care series plans to help meet the needs of these overlapping groups. It will report fundamental and applied research findings in clinically relevant, readable ways. It will provide information to teachers of primary medicine about necessary content areas such as alcoholism or the medical interview. It will also inform teachers about new teaching approaches and methods and will include some books teachers may choose to use as texts. Finally, it will publish new conceptual work about the basis of the field and the shifting paradigm of care.

This first volume is an important guide to practicing health care personnel and those preparing for such roles concerning one of the most prevalent and complex problems in primary care: alcoholism. In highly readable short chapters, the authors have managed to convey concrete useful approaches to the detection, diagnosis and treatment of alcoholism and its complications. It masterfully integrates basic research, clinical wisdom, and sound pedagogy. It is a fitting beginning for the series.

Mack Lipkin, Jr.
Series Editor

Foreword

This is an important book. It is no secret that, for decades, physicians and hospitals have tried to avoid caring for patients with problems related to alcohol consumption. This book is a milestone in the effort to reverse that trend. To become more effective, physicians and their colleagues need the kind of help provided in this volume.

The significance of alcohol-related problems is well documented; the personal, social, and economic burdens are vast. The basic problems are complex and not amenable to easy solutions. The authors respect this complexity but, on the basis of their experiences, strike an optimistic note. Without sounding overly simplistic, they relate how their clinical experiences lead them to suggest that most patients can be helped.

The book offers full recognition of the multifactorial nature of the problem and illustrates the interrelationship between the biological, psychological, social, and cultural issues which require a comprehensive approach to diagnosis and management. The various support services necessary for proper management and the physician's role in utilizing them for better patient care are presented in very practical ways. While the emphasis throughout is on the role of the primary physician, there is a general awareness of the need for an interdisciplinary approach. Thus, the need to collaborate with other health professionals and agencies, as well as with other medical specialties, is clearly shown.

The authors have performed a most valuable service in summarizing the relevant knowledge from diverse fields and gathering together the alcohol-related problems scattered among the literatures of the various professions. The focus, however, is always on the relevance for the primary care physician.

It is appropriate to note that this is not a cookbook for physicians, although it provides practical guidelines based on clinical experience of the authors. Rather, its objective is to improve the care of individual patients by enhancing the physician's understanding of the complex nature of alcoholism.

The authors are to be congratulated on the lucidity of the writing and editing. This volume demonstrates that medical writing can be readable without sacrificing accuracy. As a consequence, the book should be of value to other health professionals concerned with the care of patients with alcohol-related problems. Its ultimate impact should be the reduction of suffering and the improvement of the quality of life for alcoholic patients and their families.

Julius B. Richmond

Preface

This book is written by primary care physicians to enable other primary care practitioners to recognize and care for alcoholic patients. It is an outgrowth of the Commonwealth-Harvard Alcohol and Research Teaching Program (CHART). In 1981 this group of general internists began meeting to learn about alcoholism in order to teach their medical residents about the disease. The members of that initial group—Alan Abrams, JudyAnn Bigby, Booker Bush, Joan Savitsky, Marie Warburg, and Henrietta Barnes—have continued to care for and teach about alcoholic patients. The process of self-education clarified for us the unique role of the primary care physician in the care of patients with alcoholism.

We discovered that, although there was a wealth of information about the disease, there was no one to tell us how we, as primary care physicians, should care for alcoholic patients in our busy practices. We set out to teach ourselves by consulting experts, sharing our experiences caring for alcoholic patients, and learning how to adapt the techniques used by alcoholism counsellors to the constraints of our practices. Most of us were surprised to learn how many undiagnosed alcoholics were in our practices, and we were excited and relieved to find that we had something to offer these patients. We came to understand that the interviewing skills and long-term perspective of the practicing primary care physician were well suited to the care of many alcoholic patients.

Our initial perspective that alcoholism is "like a disease" gave way to the conviction that alcoholism is, in fact, a prototypical chronic disease. Like diabetes mellitus or multiple sclerosis, it is a disease marked by periods of remission and exacerbation which has medical, psychological, and social sequelae. There is treatment but no cure. By using alcoholism as a model, we discovered that we could teach our residents about the psychosocial aspects of a long-term illness, the importance of patient education and self-care, and the goal of improving function rather than striving for a cure. We could also teach them about alcoholism in a primary care context.

The main focus of this book is how to detect early alcoholism and how to care for patients with the disease, whether a first-time patient or one of long-standing. Although the primary locus is the physician's office, a chapter on the hospitalized patient emphasizes the importance of the primary physician in that setting. The sections on medical complications of alcoholism emphasize the subtle findings that may be present early in the disease. We have purposely not written extensively about specialized alcoholism treatment. Detailed knowledge about specific programs, which vary enormously from community to community, is less important for the primary physician than the ability to establish a diagnosis and make an effective referral. Similarly, we have chosen not to discuss the abuse of other substances. Although the increased use of both prescription and illicit drugs makes them important areas for study, it is beyond the scope of this book. However, many of the techniques that are effective for the alcoholic patient are also applicable for the drug-abusing patient in a general practice.

The reader will notice that, in general, the alcoholic patient and the physician are referred to as ''he.'' The decision to use the masculine pronoun reflects editorial convention and is not meant to affirm the stereotypes that all alcoholics and all physicians are male. Although cognizant of the debate over the terms ''recovered'' versus ''recovering,'' we have chosen to employ the more common usage, ''recovered,'' to describe the sober alcoholic.

How to Use This Book

This book illustrates approaches in making the diagnosis of alcoholism, methods for discussing it with the patient, and instituting treatment. We hope physicians will use it as a reference—whether as a quick check on the proper dosage of medication for detoxification or as a means to start a leisurely discussion on how to manage denial effectively. Each section is designed to stand alone. At the risk of redundancy, each chapter on management contains some general precepts for approaching the alcoholic patient. The reader can go to the chapter on the primary care physician's role in managing the hospitalized patient and perhaps refer to a particular medical complication without having to read the entire section on outpatient care. Although the book is relatively brief so as to be more readable, there are annotated references at the end of the book for further reading.

Acknowledgments

Several people have been instrumental in our learning about alcoholism. Stephen O'Neill, a social worker who has worked extensively in the field, helped guide the exploration of the internists' group. His familiarity with the many faces of alcoholism and his knowledge of local resources, particularly Alcoholics Anonymous, made him an invaluable member of our group. Dr. William Clark, an internist who has managed to keep one foot in general internal medicine and the other in the field of alcoholism, served as a role model. He spent hours as our preceptor discussing cases with us. He was joined by Dr. Margaret Bean-Bayog, whose insight enabled us to understand and work with the angry denial that often masks the alcoholic's anguish. Their knowledge and enthusiasm encouraged us in our study. Donald Cutler and his colleagues from the Freedom from Chemical Dependency Foundation affirmed our belief that those who have suffered with a disease have the most to teach about it. As recovered alcoholics who teach secondary school and college students about substance use and abuse, they shared with us their time, their expertise, and, most importantly, themselves. Their generosity and courage have been inspirational. The staff of the Cambridge and Somerville Program of Alcohol Rehabilitation also deserve a vote of thanks for introducing us to the world of specialized alcoholism treatment: detoxification centers, inpatient rehabilitation, and community programs.

The work that evolved into this book would not have been possible without the help of the Commonwealth Fund which generously supported our interest in alcoholism long before it was popular to do so. In particular, the Fund's President, Margaret Mahoney, and Senior Vice-President, Thomas Moloney, had the foresight to understand the important role that the general physician could play in the management of alcoholism.

We are all indebted to Marilyn Spellmeyer whose tireless editorial assistance and organization have made this book a reality.

Finally, we want to acknowledge our patients with alcoholism whose names we may forget but whose faces crowd our memory. Some we have helped, many we have not, but all of them have taught us about the disease. Although physicians will read this book, it is really written for those patients and their fellow alcoholics in the hope that these chapters will play some role in alleviating their suffering.

Henrietta N. Barnes
Mark D. Aronson
Thomas L. Delbanco

Contents

Contributors

Alan Abrams, M.D., M.P.H.
Instructor in Medicine, Department of Medicine, Harvard Medical School, Cambridge Hospital, Cambridge, MA, USA

Mark D. Aronson, M.D.
Associate Professor of Medicine, Harvard Medical School, Beth Israel Hospital, Boston, MA, USA

Henrietta N. Barnes, M.D.
Instructor in Medicine, Harvard Medical School, Massachusetts General Hospital-Chelsea Memorial Health Center, Chelsea, MA, USA

Rogelio D. Bayog, M.D.
Instructor in Psychiatry, Harvard Medical School, Brockton/West Roxbury VA Medical Center, Brockton, MA, USA

Margaret Bean-Bayog, M.D.
Assistant Professor of Psychiatry, Harvard Medical School, President American Medical Society on Alcoholism and Other Drug Dependence, Cambridge Hospital, Cambridge, MA, USA

JudyAnn Bigby, M.D.
Instructor in Medicine, Harvard Medical School, Brigham and Women's Hospital, Boston, MA, USA

Booker Bush, M.D.
Instructor in Medicine, Harvard Medical School, Beth Israel Hospital, Boston, MA, USA

Michele G. Cyr, M.D.
Assistant Professor of Medicine, Brown University Program in Medicine, Rhode Island Hospital, Providence, RI, USA

Jennifer Daley, M.D.
Assistant Professor of Medicine, Tufts University School of Medicine, New England Medical Center, Boston, MA, USA

Thomas L. Delbanco, M.D.
Associate Professor of Medicine, Harvard Medical School, Beth Israel Hospital, Boston, MA, USA

Jack Ende, M.D.
Associate Professor of Medicine, Boston University School of Medicine, University Hospital, Boston, MA, USA

Anthony W. Fox, B.Sc, M.B,
BSurg (Lond) Fellow, Clinical Pharmacology, Brigham and Women's Hospital, Boston, MA, USA

Paul A. Friedman, M.D.
Executive Director and Head, Department of Pharmacology, Merck Sharp and Dohme Research Laboratories, West Point, PA, USA

Miriam E. Griner
University of Rochester School of Medicine, Strong Memorial Hospital, Rochester, NY, USA

Paul F. Griner, M.D.
Samuel E. Durand Professor of Medicine, University of Rochester School of Medicine and Dentistry, Strong Memorial Hospital, Rochester, NY, USA

Michael A. Grodin, M.D.
Director, Program in Medical Ethics; Associate Professor of Pediatrics and Social and Behavioral Science (Ethics), Boston University Schools of Medicine and Public Health and Boston City Hospital, Boston, MA, USA

Nicholas, J. Guzman, M.D.
Fellow, Division of Nephrology and Hypertension, University of Florida, Gainesville, FL, USA

Andrea Halliday, M.D.
Resident in Surgery, Massachusetts General Hospital, Boston, MA, USA

John T. Harrington, M.D.
Professor of Medicine, Tufts University School of Medicine, Boston, Newton-Wellesley Hospital, Newton Lower Falls, MA, USA

Katherine Hesse, M.D.
Instructor in Medicine, Harvard Medical School, Mount Auburn Hospital, Cambridge, MA, USA

Ralph A. Hingson, Sc.D.
Professor in Chief, Social and Behavioral Sciences Section, Boston University School of Public Health, Boston, MA, USA

Allan Meyers, Ph.D.
Associate Professor, Department of Health Services, Boston University School of Public Health, Boston, MA, USA

Anne W. Moulton, M.D.
Assistant Professor of Medicine, Brown University Program in Medicine, Rhode Island Hospital, Providence, RI, USA

Stephen, F. O'Neill, LICSW
Clinical Instructor, Harvard Medical School, Department of Social Medicine and Health Policy, Clinical Instructor, Simmons College School of Social Work, Beth Israel Hospital, Boston, MA, USA

Julius B. Richmond, M.D.
John D. MacArthur Professor of Health Policy, Director, Division of Health Policy Research and Education, Harvard University; former Assistant Secretary for Health and Surgeon General, Department of Health and Human Services, Washington, D.C., USA

Joan Savitsky, M.D.
Instructor in Medicine, Harvard Medical School, Mount Auburn Hospital, Cambridge, MA, USA

W. Anderson Spickard, Jr., M.D.
Professor of Medicine, Vanderbilt University School of Medicine, Vanderbilt Institute for Treatment of Alcoholism (VITA), Nashville, TN, USA

Diana Chapman Walsh, Ph.D.
Associate Director, Health Policy Institute; Associate Professor, Boston University School of Public Health, Boston, MA, USA

Part I
General Concepts

1
The Epidemiology of Alcohol Abuse and the Response of Physicians

THOMAS L. DELBANCO AND HENRIETTA N. BARNES

If each primary physician addressed the issue of use and abuse of alcohol with the patients in his practice who drink moderately or heavily, the collective impact might well be felt throughout society. However, primary physicians have paid little attention to such patients.[1]

Understanding the epidemiology of alcohol use can help the practitioner judge which patients in his practice are at risk. The answer is almost everyone. Two thirds of adult Americans drink alcohol. They are about evenly divided between light drinkers (average consumption, less than one drink a day) and heavy drinkers.[2] One of three Americans reports that drinking has caused trouble in his or her own family.[3] Few primary physicians screen for signs of early difficulty even though the 9.4% prevalence of alcohol abuse or alcoholism in the general population is 1.5 times that of diabetes and hyperglycemia, for which many physicians screen routinely.

Recall, however, that normal or moderate drinkers comprise most of the patients who use alcohol. Although the incidence of alcohol-related problems is low in this group, in absolute numbers moderate drinkers will have more problems than alcoholics, despite the latter group's increased individual probability of risk.[4] These facts argue that physicians should concentrate also on the patient who drinks moderately, particularly in efforts at prevention and education.

Assessment of the drinking adult and teenager must consider cultural norms. Although American adults consume, on average, an impressive 2.7 gallons of ethanol per capita annually (the equivalent of two drinks a day), there are marked variations. In general, young adults drink more than the elderly, men consume more than women, residents of the Northeast and Pacific regions of the United States drink more than their counterparts in the South. Black and Hispanic women have high rates of abstinence, but those who do drink tend to drink heavily. Higher educational and socioeconomic status are associated with increasing alcohol consumption among whites but with lower consumption among black men.[2] Physicians should pay particular attention to a patient whose drinking behavior is atypical of his cultural context. The young white male construction worker who does not drink may have had previous problems with alcohol or may be reacting to alcoholism in his family.

Alcohol use is associated with a host of adverse events, such as suicide, motor vehicle accidents, homicides, and injuries or death secondary to falls or fire. Suicide is 30 times as common among alcoholics as among the general population. More than one half of the drivers involved in fatal accidents are intoxicated. Two thirds of all adults who drown and half who die in falling accidents or fires have been drinking.[2] Alcohol abuse is a factor in more than 10% of all deaths in the United States, roughly 200,000 per year.[5] Physicians should question patients with a history of depression or frequent trauma about their use of alcohol. Skinner et al have documented clearly the relation between multiple trauma and alcohol abuse and developed a diagnostic screening scale associating trauma with alcohol abuse.[6]

The setting of a physician's practice influences the probability of encountering patients affected by alcohol. For example, the prevalence of alcohol abuse among patients in a hospital-based practice is roughly twice that found in the population at large. Alcohol abusers represent one in every five or six patients a doctor sees, and they tend to be heavy consumers of medical care. They make more frequent office visits than nonalcoholics and require more frequent hospitalizations.[7-9] In the hospital, they use a disproportionate share of resources. Patients with a history of alcoholism, smoking, or obesity account for 10% of hospitalized patients but consume 75% of the resources.[10]

Health costs for alcohol-related problems were $15 billion in 1983. The cost to society in terms of lost productivity, traffic accidents, fires, or crime was an additional $90 billion.[11] To understand this waste in more human terms, it is possible to calculate the "potentially productive years of life lost" (PPYLL).[12] Because alcoholism is associated with up to one half of all fatal accidents and such tragedies occur most commonly in young adults, the PPYLL due to alcoholism is substantial. Moreover, these computations do not take into account the human and personal suffering of alcoholics and their families. On the brighter side, there is a small but growing body of evidence suggesting that treatment of alcoholism lowers subsequent use of health resources and lowers medical costs.[13,14]

Despite the magnitude of alcohol-related health problems, physicians have paid scant attention to these patients. Whether in a primary care, emergency unit, or hospital ward setting, less than 20% of patients with a diagnosis of alcohol abuse are identified, and the number receiving appropriate referral is even smaller.[1,15-17]

To understand why physicians have not been more active in diagnosing and managing patients with alcohol-related problems, one must look at the interlocking roles of the physician, the patient, medical education, and the health care system. Since each reflects the attitudes of society, some historical background may provide a useful context. Although Benjamin Rush conceptualized inebriety as a progressive disease in his 1786 treatise entitled "An Inquiry into the Effects of Ardent Spirits upon the Human Body and Mind"[18] his solution was to advocate abstinence and exhort church leaders to preach temperance. This moral position gathered momentum in the United States throughout the 19th century and culminated in 1919 in Prohibition, the Eighteenth Amendment to the US Constitution. Although Prohibition failed as an instrument of social control, it was highly successful in perpetuating a moral perspective on drunkenness.[19]

Since then, two models have taken a central role: the medical model and a public health model. In 1956, the American Medical Association (AMA) declared alcoholism an illness worthy of physicians' attention.[20] In the last quarter-century, organized medicine and the federal government gradually have focused more attention on the major medical implications of alcohol abuse and alcoholism, although the moral stigma attached to these problems still pervades current medical practice.[21] At the same time, there has been increased action within a public health focus, encompassing wide-ranging policies, such as increased taxation on alcoholic beverages (and thus higher prices), as in Scandinavia, or central prohibition, as in the USSR. These policies derive from the observation that mortality and incidence of cirrhosis of the liver are affected by pricing schedules or centralized governmental interdiction. In the United States, one half of all alcohol consumed is bought by the 10% of adults at particular risk. Raising the price of liquor may decrease mortality and morbidity for such drinkers, as Cook has documented in state-by-state analyses where taxation policies (and, therefore, prices) vary.[22]

When considering the practice of medicine, one must understand that alcoholic patients have a complicated impact on their physicians. The medical student's first contact with an alcoholic dying from bleeding varices or terminal cirrhosis may leave a profound sense of hopelessness. Subsequent contacts with alcoholic patients confirm that these are particularly difficult patients who often disagree with their doctor's judgment about the underlying cause of symptoms, fail to comply with advice, and miss appointments. They evoke hostility, depression, and aversion, feelings a physician must be able to tolerate and use as data in providing appropriate care.[23]

Not only may physicians find alcoholic patients emotionally difficult to care for, but they may also feel dissatisfied on an intellectual level. Many physicians would rather make a diagnosis and initiate therapy than address the ups and down of a chronic illness such as alcoholism. Furthermore, the lack of proven management strategies and outcome data frustrate rational clinical decision making. The physician must rely on his best clinical judgment, which may be clouded further by concerns about or enjoyment of his own drinking. Although recent analysis indicates that the physician is at no greater risk for alcohol abuse than the population in general,[24] the line between the healthy and unhealthy use of alcohol is a fine one.

Medical education has done little to address physicians' prejudices or to prepare them to care for alcoholics. Most of the 1% of curriculum hours devoted to teaching of substance-abuse in American medical schools are didactic lectures addressing the medical complications of alcoholism; clinical experience managing the primary problem of alcoholism is rarely offered.[25,26] In surveys of medical residents' and primary physicians' attitudes toward alcoholism, the lack of supervised clinical experience correlates with discomfort in caring for patients with alcoholism.[27,28]

A more insidious problem for the primary care physician is the dearth of role models, that is, other primary physicians who feel comfortable caring for patients with alcoholism and substance abuse. In trying to learn about alcoholism, the young physician often encounters anecdotal advice with marginal relevance to general medical practice instead of consultations based on aggregate data and carefully tested principles. This lack of consultative expertise from closely allied, dispassionate professionals may subtly dissuade the physician from increasing his interest and skills in alcoholism. The impact of role models should not be underestimated; one study of attitudes toward alcoholics found house officers more moralistic than first-year and second-year medical students.[29] Although this may simply reflect increased exposure to patients with alcoholism, one must ask why house officers are able to learn to care effectively and humanely for patients with even more devastating diseases, such as acquired immune deficiency syndrome (AIDS) and metastatic cancer.

A physician's sense that alcoholics are somehow different from other patients has been institutionalized by the health care system at large. Most care for alcoholics is provided in specialized facilities, despite the fact that more than half of these alcoholic patients who seek medical care do so from a primary care provider.[30] Recent increases in health insurance coverage for substance abuse have been a boon to specialized alcoholism treatment centers. On the other hand, the office-based physician's incentive to address alcoholism is eroded by current inequities between reasonable payment for procedural versus cognitive services. The physician has until now been paid poorly for time spent counseling the alcoholic patient and family. Thus, the impulse is to refer quickly and, at times, abdicate responsibility that might best be assumed by the primary physician.

Funding for alcohol-related research reflects the disdain of mainstream medicine for alcoholism. In terms of the proportional effects of alcoholism and cancer, for every \$1.00 spent on alcoholism, society spends \$75.00 on cancer.[21] Inadequate funding has contributed to the isolation of researchers working in an unpopular field, and it has prevented the cross-fertilization of techniques and ideas essential for high-quality investigation. It is reasonable to encourage primary physicians' interest by increasing both educational programs and research efforts. The latter would help legitimize the field, in part by generating data and techniques helpful to the practitioner. A central hypothesis of this book is that such changes will prove to be an important benefit for individual patients and society as a whole.

References

1. Kamerow DB, Pincus HA, MacDonald DI: Alcohol abuse, other drug abuse, and mental disorders in medical practice. *JAMA*, 1986;255:2054–2057.
2. *Fifth Special Report to the US Congress on Alcohol and Health*. Rockville, Md, DHHS publication No (ADM) 84-1291, 1983.

3. Fein R: *Alcohol in America: The Price We Pay.* Newport Beach, Cal, CareInstitute, 1984, p 10.
4. Moore MH, Gerstein DR (eds): *Alcohol and Public Policy: Beyond the Shadow of Prohibition*. Washington, DC, National Academy Press, 1981, p 44.
5. Public Health Service: *Healthy People: The Surgeon General's Report on Health Promotion and Disease Prevention*. DHEW publication No 79-5507. Government Printing Office, 1979.
6. Skinner HA, Holt S, Schuller R, et al: Identification of alcohol abuse using laboratory tests and a history of trauma. *Ann Intern Med* 1984;101:847–851.
7. Putnam SL: Alcoholism, morbidity and care-seeking. *Med Care* 1982;20:97–121.
8. Hallan JB: Health insurance coverage for alcoholism: A review of costs and objectives. *Alcohol Health Res World* 1981;4:16–21.
9. Hankin J, Oktay JS: Mental disorder and primary medical care: An analytical review of the literature. Rockville, Md, DHSS publication No 78-661, series D, No 5, 1979.
10. Zook CJ, Moore FD: High cost users of medical care. *N Engl J Med* 1980;302:996–1002.
11. MacDonald DI: Alcohol, Drug Abuse, and Mental Health Administration, Department of Health and Human Services. *Statement before a Hearing of the Select Committee on Children, Youth, and Families: Alcohol Abuse and Its Implications for Families*. Government Printing Office, 1985, p 34.
12. Perloff JD, LeBailly SA, Kletke PR, et al: Premature death in the United States: Years of life lost and health priorities. *J Public Health Policy* 1984;5:167–184.
13. Holder HD, Blose JO: Alcohol treatment and total health care utilization and costs. *JAMA* 1986;256:1456–1460.
14. Jones KR, Vischi TR: The impact of alcohol, drug abuse and mental health treatment on medical care utilization. *Med Care* 1979;17:1–82.
15. Bush B, Shaw S, Cleary P, et al: Screening for alcohol abuse using the CAGE questionnaire. *Am J Med* 1987;82:231–235.
16. Solomon J, Vanga N, Morgan JP, Joseph P: Emergency room physicians' recognition of alcohol misuse. *J Stud Alcohol* 1980;41(5):583–586.
17. Chappel JH, Schnoll SH: Physicians' attitudes: Effect on treatment of chemically dependent patients. *JAMA* 1977;237:2318–2319.
18. Rush B: *An Inquiry into the Effects of Ardent Spirits upon the Human Body and Mind*. The first American medical work on the effects of alcohol. Classics of the alcohol literature. *Q J Stud Alcohol* 1943;4:321–341.
19. Paredes A: The history of the concept of alcoholism, in Tarter RE, Sugerman AA (eds): *Alcoholism: Interdisciplinary Approaches to an Enduring Problem*. Reading, Mass, Addison-Wesley Publishing Co, 1976.
20. Niven RG: Alcoholism—A problem in perspective. *JAMA* 1984;252:1912–1914.
21. West LJ (ed): *Alcoholism and Related Problems: Issues of the American Public*. The American Assembly, Columbia University. Englewood Cliffs, NJ, Prentice-Hall, 1984.
22. Cook PJ: *The Economics of Alcohol Consumption and Abuse*. The American Assembly, Columbia University. Englewood Cliffs, NJ, Prentice-Hall, 1984, pp 56–77.
23. Groves JE: Taking care of the hateful patient. *N Engl J Med* 1978;298:883–887.
24. Brewster JM: Prevalence of alcoholism and other drug problems among physicians. *JAMA* 1986;255:1913–1920.
25. Helwick SA: Substance abuse in medical school: Past, present and future. *J Med Educ* 1985;60:707–711.

26. Pokorny AD, Solomon J: A follow-up survey of drug abuse and alcoholism teaching in medical schools. *J Med Educ* 1983;58:316–321.
27. Warburg MM, Cleary P, Barnes HN, et al: A survey of medical residents' attitudes toward alcoholism. *J Med Educ* 1987;62(6).
28. Rohman ME, Cleary PD, Warburg MM, et al: The response of primary care physicians to problem drinkers. *Am J Drug Alcohol Abuse* (In press).
29. Fisher JC, Mason RL, Veeley KA: Physicians and alcoholics: Effect of medical training on attitudes toward alcoholism. *J Stud Alcohol* 1975;36:949–955.
30. Shapiro S, Skinner EA, Kessler LG, et al: Utilization of health and mental health services: Three epidemiological catchment area sites. *Arch Gen Psychiatry* 1984;41:971–978.

2
Definition of Alcoholism

MARK D. ARONSON

A 66-year-old woman taking coumarin for atrial fibrillation misses multiple appointments to have her blood drawn for monitoring prothrombin time. Her physician asks frequently about her difficulty with compliance. She seems intelligent and well motivated during visits. The woman explains that she has been busy and forgets to come in for her blood test. Finally, out of frustration and concern about the danger of using the drug in an unmonitored fashion, the physician decides to discontinue the drug and the woman suffers a massive stroke. Several years later, the physician visits her in the nursing home where she resides suffering from aphasia, hemiparesis, and incontinence. It is only then that the physician learns from the woman's daughter that she is an alcoholic. She had been widowed and lived alone. She drank at night and could not recall events of the days of her life. She had been too embarrassed to tell her physician, and he, not suspecting alcoholism, failed to ask about it.

A 33-year-old engineer, married with two children, sees his physician for fatigue. His past history, review of systems, and physical examination are negative, but his social history is significant. His job is increasingly stressful, and he notes that he is leaving work a little earlier than usual because of fatigue. Further questioning reveals a pattern of drinking that suggests a problem to the physician. The patient drank heavily in college but had cut back after he completed school. He has begun to stop on the way home to drink with friends and frequently upsets his wife when he arrives home late. He has erupted in anger at her request to stop drinking and once hit her during a fight. He denies that he is an alcoholic but recognizes—with some prodding from his physician—that he might have a problem with alcohol. With his wife's and physician's help, he seeks counseling and begins abstaining from alcohol. Several months later, he notices he is no longer fatigued and tells his doctor that he realizes he is an alcoholic.

A business executive uses alcohol frequently at lunch, dinner, and in the evening. He has difficulty sleeping and uses alcohol to help him sleep at night. His employer begins noticing decreased job efficiency and warns the executive. Suspecting that his job difficulties might be due to excessive use of alcohol, the executive cuts back. When he becomes increasingly irritable, he again increases his drinking. At his wife's insistence, he sees an internist for anxiety. The physician diagnoses hypertension and stress, prescribes a sedative and suggests a less stressful job. He reassures the executive that there is nothing seriously wrong with his health.

The problem of alcoholism and alcohol abuse has many facets. Perhaps in no other area of medicine has it been as difficult to arrive at a coherent, useful, and generally acceptable definition. The patients described all had serious problems resulting from alcohol abuse; all were unable to control how much and how often they drank. The first patient had a medication-compliance problem and eventually had a stroke. The other two people described nonspecific symptoms of fatigue and stress. None of these three patients would show up in any statistics that document the impact of alcoholism on morbidity and mortality. Yet, surely, in each instance, alcohol abuse or alcoholism was the principal problem. The first patient escaped recognition by an experienced physician. The second patient's diagnosis was a surprise to the physician and the patient alike. The third patient went undiagnosed. The physician's reassurance and prescription for a sedative may, in fact, have perpetuated the problem.

What Is Alcoholism?

Most definitions of alcoholism incorporate the following dimensions: (1) large quantities of alcohol consumed over a period of years, (2) physiologic manifestations of ethanol addiction, (3) chronic loss of control over drinking, shown by an inability to stop or refrain, and (4) chronic damage to physical health or social standing resulting from sustained alcohol abuse.[1] Clark has described the fundamental lesion as "a repetitive but inconsistent and sometimes unpredictable loss of control of drinking which produces symptoms of serious dysfunction and disability, frequently including a physical addiction."[2] Yet the exact nature of alcoholism and alcohol dependency remains controversial because of sociocultural variability in the use of alcohol and the apparent overlap between normal drinking behavior and alcohol abuse.

In rural sections of France, the use of alcohol is similar to the use of coffee in the United States, that is, it is used frequently in small amounts throughout the day. People in such a society rarely become drunk but certainly can become addicted and develop medical complications, although many of the psychiatric and social consequences may not be apparent. Sociocultural differences have an enormous impact on what constitutes use and abuse of alcohol. Any user is a potential abuser, and how a particular pattern of abuse is classified depends, to a certain extent, on the cultural norm. An 18-year-old leaving a party after drinking four to five beers is not a problem drinker unless he drives a car. Yet, if that young man were in another society, his drinking might constitute abnormal drinking. Cultural differences also affect the importance placed on various adverse outcomes of alcoholism. For example, an early World Health Organization (WHO) subcommittee on alcoholism encountered difficulty because the French delegation emphasized cirrhosis, the Scandinavian group emphasized public safety, and the United States emphasized economic costs.[3]

Within the spectrum of drinkers, how does one define alcoholism? Do the people suffering from alcoholism constitute a distinct population, or are they

TABLE 2.1. The problem drinking scale (PDS).

Employer complains	Single hospital, clinic, or AA visit
Multiple job losses	3+ visits to clinics
Family and friends complain	2+ blackouts
Marital problems	Going on wagon
Multiple medical problems	Morning tremulousness and drinking
Diagnosis by clinician	Tardiness or sick leave
Alcohol-related arrest	Admits problem with control
3+ alcohol-related arrests	

Modified from Vaillant GE: *The Natural History of Alcoholism: Causes, Patterns, and Paths to Recovery.* Cambridge, Mass, Harvard University Press, 1983, p 25. Reprinted with permission.

simply the end of a spectrum that includes normal and problem drinkers? Studies from Canada suggest the latter to be the case.[4] The Lederman curve describes a unimodal distribution of alcohol intake. The smooth rather than bimodal curve implies that alcohol consumption among people with alcoholism blends into the intake of normal drinkers. Alcoholics do not apparently represent a discrete subpopulation within the entire population of drinkers.

Vaillant's long-term study of alcohol use in a sample of urban men confirms this hypothesis.[5] Rather than study alcohol consumption per se, Vaillant used scales that measured problems related to drinking. The problem drinking scale (PDS) (Table 2-1), evaluated both physiologic dependence and social deviance. Such items as employer complaints, job loss, marital problems, morning tremulousness and morning drinking, hospital or clinic visits related to alcoholism, and alcohol-related arrests were measured. Here again, there was a smooth asymptotic curve, not a bimodal one. Alcoholism appears then to be on a continuum that includes normal drinking patterns.

The Disease Concept

Nevertheless, alcoholism is not normal, and the concept that alcoholism is a disease[6] has clear precedent. Hypertension provides an analogy; the level of blood pressure is distributed in a unimodal manner in the population, with those individuals at one end of the curve labeled as hypertensive. Just as the adverse sequelae of hypertension are related to the height of the blood pressure, so too are the adverse consequences of alcohol abuse and alcoholism correlated with the increased intake of alcohol.

Understanding alcoholism as a disease is useful in caring for patients with drinking problems. First, it enables physicians to use familiar techniques to make a diagnosis, form a treatment plan, provide patient education, and discuss a prognosis. It helps differentiate alcoholism from a bad habit (despite Szacz' assertions to the contrary[7]) or a moral weakness from lack of will power and legitimizes interventions, such as Alcoholics Anonymous (AA) and disulfiram. Perhaps most importantly, it obligates the physician to address the problem of alcoholism and, in a nonjudgmental way, confront the patient with the truth about his diagnosis. The disease is alcoholism; if untreated, it can progress; it is often fatal. However, therapy is available, and the patient can be helped.

The Diagnosis of Alcoholism

What then constitutes the diagnosis of alcoholism? Several organizations have attempted to define alcohol abuse and alcoholism. The National Council on Alcoholism (NCA) developed criteria for the diagnosis of alcoholism that incorporate many of the physiologic and medical consequences of alcoholism.[8] The NCA and the Committee on Definitions of the American Medical Society on Alcoholism defined alcoholism as a "chronic, progressive and potentially fatal disease . . . characterized by tolerance and physical dependency or pathologic organ changes or both—all these direct or indirect consequences of the alcohol ingested."[9]

The American Psychiatric Association's *Diagnostic and Statistical Manual -III (DSM-III)*[10] attempts to make diagnoses based on clinical observations rather than theoretical or etiologic grounds. The *DSM-III* (Table 2-2) provides a useful definition of alcohol abuse and alcohol dependency (what others refer to as "alcoholism"). By alcohol abuse, the DSM refers to patterns of pathologic use, for instance, morning drinking, inability to cut down or stop drinking, and impairment of social and occupational functioning caused by the pattern of pathologic use. They also imply by this definition that the problem has lasted for at least one month. Alcohol dependency is a more severe form of the problem and corresponds with earlier definitions that focus on late-stage disease, such as the NCA criteria.[8] Here, there is not only the pattern of pathologic use of alcohol and social and occupational difficulties resulting from the alcohol use but also symptoms of physical addiction manifested by either tolerance or withdrawal.

WHO has developed the concept of an alcohol dependency syndrome, a provisional description of which was published in the *British Medical Journal* in 1976.[11] The cardinal features include narrowing of the drinking pattern, salience of drink-seeking behavior, increased tolerance to alcohol, repeated withdrawal symptoms, release-avoidance of withdrawal, subjective awareness of compulsion to drink, and recurrence of symptoms after relapse. WHO also proposes a separate classification of alcohol-related disabilities, for example, a person may suffer consequences of alcoholism, such as automobile accidents or cirrhosis, without actually developing the dependency syndrome.[12] These proposals by WHO allow for a broader understanding of the disorder, and one could fit any of the patients described earlier in this chapter into such a scheme.

Vaillant has conceptualized three stages of alcoholism: (1) the asymptomatic drinker, (2) the alcohol abuser, and (3) the alcohol dependent.[13] The asymptomatic drinker may be a heavy drinker but has not as yet suffered the adverse

TABLE 2.2. Definitions: Alcohol abuse and alcohol dependency.

The essential feature of alcohol abuse is a pattern of pathologic use for at least a month that causes impairment in social or occupational functioning.

The essential features of alcohol dependency are either a pattern of pathologic alcohol use or impairment in social or occupational functioning due to alcohol, and either tolerance or withdrawal. Dependency has also been called alcoholism.

Course

When abuse or dependency develops, it is usually within the first 5 years after regular drinking is established. Heavy drinking in adolescence (before age 16) is particularly likely to be associated with later problems.

Although alcohol dependency and abuse can continue into old age, they may remit with aging, sometimes in response to the development of physical complications. Occasional drinking with rare or no episodes of intoxication does occur in some persons with a clear prior history of alcohol dependency. Therefore, drinking that is currently moderate should not be considered evidence for the absence of alcohol dependency in the past.

There are three main patterns of chronic pathologic alcohol use. The first is regular daily intake of large amounts; the second is regular heavy drinking limited to weekends. These two patterns are included in the fifth-digit subtype "Continuous." The third pattern is long periods of sobriety interspersed with binges of daily heavy drinking lasting for weeks or months. This pattern corresponds to the fifth-digit subtype "Episodic."

Familial pattern

Alcohol abuse and dependency are more common among family members than in the general population. Evidence of a genetic factor is the increased prevalence of alcohol dependency in the early-adopted offspring of parents with the disorder.

Diagnostic Criteria for Alcohol Abuse

A. Pattern of pathologic alcohol use: Need for daily use of alcohol for adequate functioning, inability to cut down or stop drinking, repeated efforts to control or reduce excess drinking by going on the wagon (periods of temporary abstinence) or restricted drinking to certain times of the day, binges (remaining intoxicated throughout the day for at least 2 days), occasional consumption of a fifth of spirits (or its equivalent in wine or beer), amnesic periods for events occurring while intoxicated (blackouts), continuation of drinking despite a serious physical disorder that the person knows is exacerbated by alcohol use; drinking of nonbeverage alcohol.

B. Impairment in social or occupational functioning due to alcohol use: eg, violence while intoxicated, absence from work, loss of job, legal difficulties (arrest for intoxicated behavior, traffic accidents while intoxicated), arguments or difficulties with family or friends because of excessive alcohol use.

C. Duration of disturbance of at least one month.

Diagnostic Criteria for Alcohol Dependency

A. Either a pattern of pathologic alcohol use or impairment in social or occupational functioning due to alcohol use:

Pattern of pathologic alcohol use: Need for daily use of alcohol for adequate functioning, inability to cut down or stop drinking, repeated efforts to control or reduce excess drinking by going on the wagon (periods of temporary abstinence) or restricted drinking to certain times of the day, binges (remaining intoxicated throughout the day for at least two days), occasional consumption of a fifth of spirits (or its equivalent in wine or beer), amnesic periods for events occurring while intoxicated (blackouts), continuation of drinking despite a serious physical disorder that the person knows is exacerbated by alcohol use, drinking of nonbeverage alcohol.

Impairment in social or occupational functioning due to alcohol use: eg, violence while intoxicated, absence from work, loss of job, legal difficulties (arrest for intoxicated behavior, traffic accidents while intoxicated), arguments or difficulties with family or friends because of excessive alcohol use.

TABLE 2.2. (*Continued*).

B. Either tolerance or withdrawal:
Tolerance: Need for markedly increased amounts of alcohol to achieve the desired effort or markedly diminished effect with regular use of the same amount.
Withdrawal: development of alcohol withdrawal (eg, morning shakes and malaise relieved by drinking) after cessation of or reduction in drinking.

Adapted from American Psychiatric Association: *Diagnostic and Statistical Manual of Mental Disorders*, ed 3. Washington, DC, American Psychiatric Association, 1980. Reprinted with permission.

consequences of drinking. This drinker (referring to an adult male) consumes roughly two ounces of ethanol per day or approximately four cans of beer. This stage may go on without change over many years, but it may evolve into alcohol abuse. The alcohol abuser may suffer from the medical, legal, and social consequences of alcoholism, for example, automobile accidents, falls, blackouts, and marital difficulties. Usually intake exceeds three ounces of alcohol per day (seven or more drinks per 24 hours). Perhaps one third of these people do not evolve further. Another third return to asymptomatic drinking, and about one third to one half evolve into alcohol dependency, or alcoholism. Such a person has repetitive loss of control of drinking. Withdrawal symptoms are common and eventually require treatment. In perhaps the best longitudinal study of the natural history of alcoholism, Vaillant has shown how various definitions and scales evaluating alcoholism support this concept. He argues that a strict analysis of individual symptoms does not, by itself, diagnose alcoholism but that it is the number, frequency, and variety of these adverse sequelae that define alcoholism.[5] In his analysis, it mattered little if one measured medical or social sequelae.

It is apparent that it is an arbitrary decision where one defines the cutoff for alcoholism on any of the scales referred to or on the Lederman curve. Alcohol abuse appears to lie on a continuum of severity[14] and may manifest itself in a variety of ways. As it becomes more severe, it becomes less plastic[11] and abstinence becomes more difficult. In addition, the syndrome of withdrawal and the well-recognized physiologic consequences (Part III) become more prominent and obvious. A simple conceptualization is that most of the alcohol in the world is consumed by normal drinkers, but most of the adverse sequelae are suffered by a small number of people (perhaps 3 to 6 percent of the United States population). These people individually consume more alcohol than most normal drinkers, and they suffer the largest number of adverse sequelae. They are the people (patients) whom physicians call alcoholics.

Discussion

Alcoholism is a common problem that has classic clinical features in its advanced stages. As can be seen from the cases cited at the start of this chapter, the disease can elude diagnosis (while patients manifest nonspecific symptoms) in the early stages. Patients may have medical, legal, or social difficulties. Physicians must appreciate the fact that alcoholism is part of a continuum that includes normal drinking at one end of the spectrum. Where alcoholism starts on the spectrum is somewhat arbitrary, but the criteria and scales presented in this chapter may be useful in making decisions about individual patients. First, however, the diagnosis must be considered and asked about. If alcoholism is recognized and treated in its early stages, the more severe consequences of heavy and prolonged alcohol consumption can be avoided.

References

1. Armor DJ, Polich JM, Stambul HB: *Alcoholism and Treatment*. New York, John Wiley and Sons, 1978, p 11.
2. Clark WD: Alcoholism: Blocks to diagnosis and treatment. *Am J Med* 1981;71:275–286.
3. Heath DB: Sociocultural variants in alcoholism, in Pattison EM, Kaufman E (eds): *Encyclopedic Handbook of Alcoholism*. New York, Gardner Press, 1982, pp 426–439.
4. Schmidt W, Popham RE: The single distribution theory of alcohol consumption. *Q J Stud Alcohol* 1978;39:400–419.
5. Vaillant GE: *The Natural History of Alcoholism: Causes, Patterns, and Paths to Recovery*. Cambridge, Mass, Harvard University Press, 1983, pp 15–44.
6. Jellinek EM: *Disease Concept of Alcoholism*. New Haven, Hillhouse Press, 1960.
7. Szacz T: Bad habits are not diseases. *Lancet* 1972;2:83–84.
8. Criteria Committee. National Council on Alcoholism: Criteria for the diagnosis of alcoholism. *Ann Intern Med* 1972;77:249–258.
9. Seixas FA, Blume S, Cloud LA, et al: Definition of alcoholism. *Ann Intern Med* 1976;85:764.
10. *Diagnostic and Statistical Manual of Mental Disorders*, ed 3. Washington, DC, American Psychiatric Association, 1980, p 70.
11. Edwards G, Gross MM: Alcohol dependence: Provisional description of a clinical syndrome. *Br Med J* 1976;1:1058–1061.
12. Royal College of Psychiatrists: *Alcohol and Alcoholism*. New York, Free Press, 1979.
13. Vaillant GE: *The Natural History of Alcoholism: Causes, Patterns, and Paths to Recovery*. Cambridge, Mass, Harvard University Press, 1983, pp 309–310.
14. Skinner HA, Holt S, Israel Y: Early identification of alcohol abuse: Critical issues and psychosocial indicators for a composite index. *Can Med Assoc J* 1981;124: 1141–1152.

3
The Etiology and Natural History of Alcoholism

HENRIETTA N. BARNES

JL, a middle-aged real estate broker, is brought to the emergency room for evaluation of possible internal injuries following a motor vehicle accident. He is under arrest for driving while intoxicated. Alternately belligerent and morose, he states that recent marital difficulties have "driven him to drink," just like his father before him. Other than intoxication, physical examination is remarkable for an enlarged liver, with liver function tests compatible with alcoholic hepatitis. After telling Mr L that if he does not stop drinking he will die of liver disease, the emergency room physician walks away shaking her head about another hopeless alcoholic.

Is Mr L's condition really so hopeless? Must he either abstain from alcohol or face certain death? Is his problem the result of hostile sociopathic tendencies and a disrupted family life? Does he suffer from a disease or just a bad habit with disastrous medical, psychologic, and socioeconomic consequences?

Our experiences as physicians confirm many of the myths about the causes and development of alcoholism. Single encounters with alcoholic patients, like the man described above, give rise to associations between alcohol and behavior that are often correct. However, assumptions about causality may be misleading. The goal of this chapter is to summarize what is known about the etiology and natural history of alcoholism, addressing the following clinical questions:

1. What are the risk factors for alcoholism?
2. Is there a typical prealcoholic personality?
3. How does a person develop alcoholism?
4. What is the course of the disease and its prognosis?
5. Does treatment affect the course of the disease?

The answers depend on where one looks. The breadth of alcoholism, affecting some 3% to 6% of adult Americans, and its depth, extending over decades, make it impossible for any one observer to encompass the problem. The reviewer must acknowledge the unique advantages and limitations of different perspectives. The literature in sociology provides a background picture of normal drinking practices, cultural differences, and predisposing factors, such as heredity, but it does not address the development of the disease. Clinical studies, especially prospective studies, have much to say about the development of alcoholism in a population of alcoholics but little about the experience of one alcoholic patient. Case studies can provide that individual context. Finally, psychologic models, although unproven, provide a framework for understanding how alcoholism may develop.

There are limitations in the research on alcoholism. First, because the disease of alcoholism itself distorts the recollection of past events, retrospective data are necessarily suspect. Second, most study populations have been composed of middle-aged, white men with severe disease—hardly representative of women, minority, adolescent, or elderly alcoholics. Finally, unacknowledged bias of two types is common: (1) inadequate length of follow-up and (2) selective study populations, for example, sociopaths or alcoholics already in treatment.

Risk Factors for Alcoholism

Risk factors for alcoholism fall into three categories: family history, ethnic background, and occupation or social milieu. These three factors describe the social fabric of most people's lives. As such, it is difficult to ascertain the relative weight of these risk factors, but the composite picture enables the clinician to gauge a patient's risk for alcohol abuse. Information about risk factors is easily obtained as part of a routine medical history.

Family History

A family history of alcohol abuse in two or more relatives increases the risk of developing alcoholism by a factor of three.[1] Whether this difference is the result of heredity or environment needs to be answered.

The genetic evidence comes from studies designed to separate nature from nurture. Comparisons of identical and fraternal twins[2,3] indicate that identical twins have a higher concordance for drinking behavior and possibly alcoholism. Adoption and half-sibling studies have more clearly separated heredity and environment. In comparing Danish children of alcoholics (whether raised by their own alcoholic parent or adopted) to a control population of children without an alcoholic parent (but with similar circumstances of adoption), Goodwin found that sons of alcoholics had four times the risk of developing alcoholism, whether raised by their biologic parents or by nonalcoholic foster parents.[4] Worthy of note is the fact that the sons of alcoholics did not differ significantly from the control group in any other variable designed to measure psychopathology, drinking behavior, or use of other drugs. Shuckit's study of half-siblings of alcoholics corroborates Goodwin's and Vaillant's findings: half-siblings with an alcoholic biologic parent in common were three times more likely to develop alcoholism than those half-siblings without a common alcoholic parent, whether they were raised in an alcoholic environment or not.[5]

A disruptive childhood environment, long considered a predictor of future alcoholism, was not an independent risk factor when parental alcoholism was controlled for in Vaillant's study of disadvantaged urban men—the Core City sample.[1] A similar finding that alcohol abuse was independent of childhood environment in a more socially privileged cohort of college men suggests that these results may be generalizable.[6]

Ethnic Background

Genetic susceptibility, the role of alcohol in the society, and culturally accepted drinking practices fall under the heading of ethnic background. Although evidence of racial differences in the ability to metabolize alcohol exists—most notably, many Orientals have an unpleasant reaction to small amounts of alcohol[7]—there is no clear evidence that a genetic predisposition on a racial level (as opposed to a familial level) increases the risk of developing alcoholism.

Cultures that teach children to use alcohol in the context of the family, condone the moderate use of alcohol as a beverage with food, and discourage public intoxication have lower rates of alcoholism. Cross-cultural studies are very difficult to interpret because of many confounding variables, such as type and availability of alcohol or differences in reporting alcohol use. Vaillant's Core City sample, with 61% of the subjects' parents foreign-born, fortuitously controls for many of these variables. Men of Irish and other Northern European backgrounds had similar risks for alcoholism, which was five to six times that of men of Mediterranean background. However, the risk of problem drinking was similar in all ethnic groups.[1]

Occupation and Social Milieu

High rates of alcoholism are found in such disparate occupational groups as bartenders, seamen, insurance brokers, and physicians. Characteristics found in these occupations include accessibility to alcohol during work hours, social pressure from co-workers to drink, separation from or disruption of normal family and social routines, minimal supervision, and intrinsic job-related stresses.[8] Additionally, these types of occupations may attract people with a predisposition to problems with alcohol.

A person's immediate social network will affect (or reflect) his drinking practices. Vaillant notes that many young heavy drinkers in his Core City sample modified their drinking practices when they married and changed their social networks.[1] In a larger social context, ready availability of alcohol—low cost relative to other goods or a low legal drinking age—and cultural preference for high-proof alcoholic beverages tend to increase the risk of alcohol abuse.

In summary, the identification of multiple risk factors for alcohol abuse is consistent with its multifactorial etiology. Obtaining information on family history, cultural background, and occupation will enable physicians to offer advice about the risk of developing alcoholism and may help patients modify some of those risks.

Is There a Typical Pre-alcoholic Personality?

Any clinician can describe the typical alcoholic: a person who is anxious and depressed, emotionally inconsistent, and irresponsible, someone who manifests hostility and sociopathic tendencies and has difficulty with interpersonal relationships. Psychologic and psychiatric studies confirm the practitioner's impressions[9] but leave unanswered the question of whether these personality characteristics predate alcoholism or are the consequence of it.

The literature suggests that there is no evidence for a characteristic premorbid personality for future alcoholics. The personality profile of college freshmen who later developed alcoholism showed no obvious deviation from the norm when they were tested in college, but test results when they were in alcoholism treatment years later reflect the personality traits outlined above.[10] One third of Vaillant's college sophomores who later developed alcohol abuse were rated in the top category for psychologic health. In fact, the predictors of future mental illness in Vaillant's Core City sample (childhood emotional problems and the absence of boyhood competence and strong childhood environment) did not increase the risk of future alcohol abuse.[1]

The one area that demands closer scrutiny is the relationship between alcoholism and sociopathy. Is abuse of alcohol just one expression of an underlying antisocial personality, or do alcoholics manifest sociopathic tendencies as a result of their alcoholism? Or perhaps there is a common etiologic factor underlying both alcoholism and sociopathy.[11] In comparing the alcoholics and sociopaths in his Core City group, Vaillant notes a similar pattern of alcohol dependence and antisocial behavior in both groups. However, the sociopaths were more likely to begin abusing alcohol at a younger age, to manifest a more disrupted life (multiple arrests, hospitalizations, and job losses), and to deny that alcohol was a problem. A common antecedent of sociopathy and alcoholism noted by Vaillant was the presence of hyperactivity, and several other authors have suggested that this may play a role in the development of alcoholism.[12]

How Does a Person Develop Alcoholism?

Why someone continues to drink excessively when there are known adverse consequences is a question that frequently plagues physicians. Understanding how a person develops dependence on alcohol can begin to answer that question. Although it is impossible to predict who of those who are at risk for alcoholism will actually develop the disease, once the process has started there is a fairly characteristic pattern of psychologic and behavioral events.

Drinking alcoholic beverages is a learned behavior. Initial drinking experiences teach an individual that drinking alcohol provides a positive mood swing that is dose related.[13] Normal drinkers learn to seek that mood swing for recreational enjoyment, for sedative effects, or for the relief of tension and anxiety. Early drinking experience often involves occasional episodes of intoxication. The drinker's euphoria may be followed by unpleasant effects (nausea, vomiting, feeling hungover) or regret about behavior while still intoxicated. As drinking habits mature, the individual usually moderates his intake to a level that maximizes the positive and minimizes the negative effects of drinking.

A person who is developing dependence on alcohol apparently does not have the feedback mechanism that leads to moderate drinking. Whether this defect is psychologic or physiologic is unclear, and no definite biochemical defect has been identified. Most likely, the etiology is multifactorial and may not be the same for all people with alcoholism.[14,15] As a person continues to have episodes of excessive intake, there are more negative consequences. Initially these are behavioral: embarrassing behavior while intoxicated, increased tension with spouse and family, decreased interest in activities that do not include drinking. Similar to the normal drinker, the future alcoholic attempts to moderate his intake (as if his drinking were completely volitional), but once alcoholism develops, drinking is in part beyond his control. Repeated failure to maintain control over drinking undermines the drinker's self-respect and amplifies the pain and guilt associated with the negative effects of drinking.[16]

Since the drinker has learned that alcohol relieves tension and anxiety, he turns to alcohol to alleviate his pain and guilt. Alcohol becomes the solution, not the problem. The alcoholic now faces a conflict between the need to drink and knowledge of the adverse effects of drinking. The psychologic solution is to deny that drinking has negative effects. Denial can be defined as a psychologic defense against a reality that is too painful to bear.[17] For the alcoholic, the idea that he should give up alcohol, coupled with the knowledge that he has not been able to stop, is so intolerable that the harmful effects of drinking are denied. Denial enables the drinker to continue drinking and to maintain some modicum of self-esteem.

The alcoholic uses other psychologic defenses to buttress denial. The following vignettes will be familiar to most clinicians and illustrate the alcoholic's use of rationalization, projection, and minimization.

My clients expect me to have a few drinks with them when we're discussing business over lunch.
You'd drink, too, if your husband was always nagging you about the housework.
Well, I only had one drink, and one never hurt anyone.

Although denial is primarily a psychologic mechanism, there is a large organic component. Repeated use of alcohol impairs intellectual and emotional function secondary to its toxic effects on the central nervous system (CNS). Chronic abuse of alcohol induces blackouts, which are periods of amnesia for events and behavior while intoxicated. Alcohol-induced depression and impaired judgment prevent the alcoholic person from using his rational coping skills to address his alcoholism.[16]

This psychodynamic model of the development of alcoholism and denial is drawn from the observation of experienced clinicians. It describes a common pattern in many reported case histories,[1,16,18] although the course and progression of the disease may vary enormously.

What Is the Course of the Disease?

Classic teaching about alcoholism describes the disease as an inexorable downward progression leading either to abstinence or death. More recent long-term studies indicate that the course of alcoholism in a cohort of alcoholics is, in fact, quite varied[1,19] and that the course for a particular person may be even more variable. Although the classic description of alcoholism has assumed mythic proportions, it is still a useful basis for an initial understanding of the disease.

Progressive Disease

The progressive nature of the disease has been articulated best by Jellinek.[20] His model, based on the stories of 2,000 male alcoholics associated with Alcoholics Anonymous (AA), describes four phases of alcohol addiction. In the initial *prealcoholic symptomatic phase*, the alcoholic learns to drink to relieve tension and develops a tolerance to alcohol. This stage of operant conditioning usually lasts months to two years. The alcoholic then begins to experience blackouts and enters the *prodromal phase*, characterized by changes in drinking behavior (surreptitious drinking, gulping drinks, preoccupation with alcohol, and increasing guilt about the use of alcohol). Toward the end of this phase the alcoholic begins to experience loss of control over drinking. Jellinek makes a clear distinction between the alcoholic's ability to control the initiation of a drinking episode and the difficulty in maintaining control once drinking has started. The next *crucial phase* encompasses the psychologic and behavioral changes that occur as the alcoholic adapts to the addiction. Jellinek describes the alcoholic's rationalizations, grandiosity, aggressive outbursts, and remorse. Life now centers around alcohol – maintaining a supply, drinking in the morning, and occasionally attempting abstinence. Prolonged periods of intoxication are rare until the final stage of *chronic intoxication*, which includes the marked deterioration of the alcoholic's psychologic functioning and physical health, paralleled by the dissolution of his usual social network. At this point, the alcoholic is "spontaneously accessible to treatment. Nevertheless, his obsessive drinking continues as he does not see a way out."[20]

This progressive course applies to approximately three quarters of the Core City alcoholics in Vaillant's sample,[1] half of whom achieved abstinence. A four year follow-up study of the sample in the original Rand report,[21] which looked at the outcome of approximately 500 men seen at outpatient alcohol treatment centers, apparently confirms Valliant's figures. Seventy-five percent of the alcoholics fit Jellinek's model of progressive disease; about two thirds of them drank alcoholically and one third were abstinent for at least a year.[19] In contrast, over an eight year period of follow-up, 95% of alcoholics seeking inhospital treatment for alcoholism manifested the progressive course described by Jellinek.[1] One could surmise that at the other (healthier) end of the spectrum, a population of early-stage alcoholics would show much more variation in their disease, with many more people falling into the categories of (1) nonproblem or asymptomatic drinkers and (2) stable, nonprogressive alcohol abusers. All these categories are somewhat fluid, and any one alcoholic may move in and out of a category at different times.

Nonproblem or Asymptomatic Drinking

The alcoholics who have returned to nonproblem drinking comprise about 16% to 18% of Vaillant's Core City sample and the Rand sample, although percentages from treatment settings are usually lower.[1,19] Nonproblem or asymptomatic drinking is not normal social drinking—many of these drinkers must exercise constraint (type of beverage, places and hours of drinking) in order to avoid problems. The amount of alcohol consumed may vary from a drink less often than once a month to daily consumption of several drinks.[19] Vaillant describes one man who would go to a bar only on Saturday after 10:30 PM, knowing that the bar's closing at midnight would limit his consumption.[1] Whether these alcoholics have a different kind of alcoholism or whether they have a less severe form of the disease described by Jellinek is not known. It is clear that they differ significantly from their counterparts who have continued to experience problems with alcohol. Men who returned to asymptomatic drinking were less likely to be physically dependent on alcohol, had experienced fewer alcohol-related problems (job loss, medical problems), described a shorter duration of loss of control drinking, and were less likely to have received any treatment for alcoholism.[1]

Stable, Nonprogressive Drinking

The "atypical alcoholic," to use Vaillant's phrase, who abuses alcohol without any apparent progression of disease, represents only a small fraction of patients with alcoholism. Generally he is a binge-drinker who manifests relatively few alcohol-related problems. This does not imply that no adverse consequences are experienced but rather that an equilibrium between alcohol abuse and the rest of his life has been established.

Relapse

The simplification inherent in this discussion suggests that the course of alcoholism is unidirectional, whether to abstinence, nonproblem drinking, or continued alcohol abuse. In fact, relapse is common. Most alcoholics cross the line from drinking to abstinence many times in the course of their disease. Only 7% of the Rand group maintained a stable abstinence over four years, but an additional 21% had experienced at least six months of abstinence.[19] From the clinician's perspective, knowing who is susceptible to relapse and why can be very helpful in working with alcoholic patients. Relapse results from the interplay of individual and external factors. The obvious causes, and the ones often cited by patients, are external stresses: death in the family, divorce, change or loss of job. A disrupted social network does put the recovering alcoholic at increased risk of relapse. More subtle, and perhaps more significant, are internal factors in which psychologic conditioning plays a more important role than psychopathology. Emotional cues that trigger drinking behavior and the expectation that alcohol will help the situation and result in certain behavior are part of the addictive process and are independent of the pharmacology of ethanol.[1]

The different courses of alcoholism should not obscure the fact that for most alcoholics it is a chronic disease with exacerbations and remissions. It carries a mortality 2.5 to 3 times that expected for any given age.[22] In general, the early deaths represent the alcoholics who continue to abuse alcohol, but the mortality of those who have returned to nonproblem drinking is higher than that of the abstainers.[19] Although most of the excess mortality is secondary to alcohol-related disease, cardiovascular disease makes a significant contribution in older age groups.

Does Treatment Affect the Course of the Disease?

There are two ways to address this question. One is to review outcome studies of the different types of treatment, and the other is to study alcoholics who have recovered and try to identify what factors were important in their achieving abstinence.

The first pathway yields some interesting information, but it is fraught with problems. Limited follow-up, measured in months, may demonstrate good results that are not borne out by longer periods of observation. For example, in the initial Rand report, 70% of their sample were in remission (some improvement in drinking behavior) at 18 months, but in four years, that figure dropped to 46%.[19,21] In longer periods of follow-up, it is all but impossible to control for other forms of treatment, such as AA. Finally, different criteria for successful outcomes, ranging from a few months of abstinence to an improvement in social function, have made any comparison of results problematic.

Reviews of treatment[1,23,24] are discouraging. Recovery rates with treatment are not significantly better than the rate for spontaneous recovery. However, they show that recovery is more closely associated with patient characteristics than with the particular type of treatment.[23] Premorbid social stability, particularly marital status and employment, is associated with a positive outcome. Although this association could be dismissed as a tautology indicating only that healthier people do better, it also suggests that early intervention in alcoholism may lead to a better outcome. In a provocative study, Edwards et al suggest that a three-hour session of treatment and advice may be as efficacious as intensive inpatient treatment.[25] By extrapolation, even a brief intervention by a busy clinician may have some therapeutic value.

Whereas alcohol specialists may debate the relative merits of different treatment programs, less than one third of the abstinent alcoholics in Vaillant's Core City sample credit formal alcohol treatment (other than AA) as an important factor in their stopping drinking.[1] The nontreatment factors fall into four categories: substitute dependency, behavior modification, enhanced hope and self-esteem, and new social stability. The substitute dependencies usually revolved around some form of compulsive behavior, use of another chemical, or meditation. Modification of behavior was likely to result from an internal negative consequence, such as acute medical problems from drinking, rather than external coercion. The major source of hope and improved self-esteem was AA, although involvement in religion played a prominent role for some. Social stability usually involved the establishment of a new love relationship predicated on the alcoholic's abstinence.

Vaillant's work indicates that the turning point between active alcoholism and sobriety is not a mystical occurrence. The course of the disease is clearly susceptible to certain pressures, although these may reflect more the alcoholic's ability to heal himself than a specific treatment program. Certainly, in the short run, treatment for alcoholism can decrease morbidity whether one looks at it in terms of human suffering or economic cost.

Implications for the Practitioner

Although the course, manifestation, and prognosis of alcoholism are extremely variable, the pessimism of the emergency room physician in the case presented at the beginning of the chapter does not seem warranted. Some alcoholics recover; many improve. If the goal with alcoholic patients, as with people who suffer from other chronic diseases, is to palliate suffering, lengthen periods of remission, and improve function, knowledge of the natural history of the disease will allow physicians to respond appropriately to their alcoholic patients. Knowledge about risk factors enables clinicians to educate patients about healthy drinking practices and the warning signs of hazardous drinking. Understanding that alcoholism is more often the cause than the result of psychologic and behavioral problems should prompt physicians to address the issue of alcoholism directly. The establishment of reasonable goals for alcoholic patients will allow physicians to treat such patients with hope and respect. In the conclusion to his book, *The Natural History of Alcoholism: Causes, Patterns, and Paths to Recovery*, Vaillant says, "somewhat paradoxically, recognition of our limited ability to alter the course of the disease may lead to improved care, not chaos."[1]

References

1. Vaillant GE: *The Natural History of Alcoholism: Causes, Patterns, and Paths to Recovery.* Cambridge, Mass, Harvard Univ Press, 1983.

2. Kaij L: *Studies on the Etiology and Sequels of Abuse of Alcohol*, thesis. University of Lund, Sweden, 1960.
3. Partanen J, Bruun K, Markkanen T: *Inheritance of Drinking Behavior: A Study on Intelligence, Personality, and Use of Alcohol in Adult Twins*. Helsinki, Finland, Finnish Foundation for Alcohol Studies, 1966, pp 14–59.
4. Goodwin DW: Alcoholism and heredity. *Arch Gen Psychiatry* 1979;36:57–61.
5. Schuckit MA: A study of alcoholism in half-siblings. *Am J Psychiatry* 1972;128:1132–1136.
6. Vaillant GE: Natural history of male psychological health. II. Some antecedents of healthy adult adjustment. *Arch Gen Psychiatry* 1974;31:15–22.
7. Ewing JA, Rouse BA, Pellizar ED: Alcohol sensitivity and ethnic background. *Am J Psychiatry* 1974;131:206–210.
8. Plant ML: *Drinking Careers*. London, Tabistock, 1979.
9. Blum EM: Psychoanalytic views of alcoholism: A review. *Q J Stud Alcohol* 1966;27:259–299.
10. Kammeier ML, Hoffman H, Loper RG: Personality characteristics of alcoholics as college freshmen and at the time of treatment. *Q J Stud Alcohol* 1973;34:390–399.
11. Schuckit MA: Alcoholism and sociopathy—Diagnostic confusion. *Q J Stud Alcohol* 1973;34:157–164.
12. Tarter RE: Minimal brain dysfunction as an etiological predisposition to alcoholism, in Meyer RE, et al (eds): *Evaluation of the Alcoholic: Implications for Research, Theory, and Treatment*. NIAAA Monograph Series, 1981.
13. Johnson VE: *I'll Quit Tomorrow*. New York; Harper and Row, 1975.
14. Paredes A, Hood WR, Seymour H, Gollob M: Loss of control in alcoholism: An investigation of the hypothesis, with experimental findings. *Q J Stud Alcohol* 1973;34:1146–1161.
15. Ludwig AM, Benfeldt F, Wikler A, et al: "Loss of control" in alcoholics. *Arch Gen Psychiatry* 1978;35:370–373.
16. Bean MH: Denial and the psychological complications of alcoholism, in Bean MH, Zinberg NE (eds.): *Dynamic Approaches to the Understanding and Treatment of Alcoholism*. New York; Free Press, 1981, pp 55–96.
17. Paredes A: Denial, deceptive maneuvers and consistency in behavior of alcoholics. *Ann NY Acad Sci* 1973;233:23–31.
18. Clark WD: Alcoholism: Blocks to diagnosis and treatment. *Am J Med* 1981;71: 275–286.
19. Polich JM, Armor DJ, Braiker HB: *The Course of Alcoholism: Four Years after Treatment*. New York; John Wiley and Sons, 1981.
20. Jellinek EM: Phases of alcohol addiction. *Q J Stud Alcohol*. 1952;13(4):673–684.
21. Armor DG, Polich JM, Stambul HB: *Alcoholism and Treatment*. New York; John Wiley and Sons, 1978.
22. *Fifth Special Report to the US Congress on Alcohol and Health*. Rockville, Md, DHHS Publication No (ADM)84-1291, 1983.
23. Baekeland F: Evaluation of treatment methods in chronic alcoholism, in Kissin B, Begleiter H (eds.): *The Biology of Alcoholism*. New York; Plenum Press, 1977, vol 5: *Treatment and Rehabilitation on the Chronic Alcoholic*, pp 385–440.
24. Emrick CD: A review of psychologically oriented treatment of alcoholism. II. The relative effectiveness of different treatment approaches and the effectiveness of treatment versus no treatment. *J Stud Alcohol* 1974;36:88–109.
25. Edwards G, Orford J, Egert S, et al: Alcoholism: A controlled trial of "treatment" and "advice." *J Stud Alcohol* 1977;38:1004–1031.

Part II
The Clinical Pharmacology of Alcohol

4
The Clinical Pharmacology of Alcohol

ANTHONY W. FOX, NICOLAS J. GUZMAN,
and PAUL A. FRIEDMAN

There is a vast amount of literature about the pharmacology of alcohol. However, there are limitations to the clinical applicability of much of the information, since many of the studies reported are in animals, and extrapolation from animal models to humans can be misleading. Further, most of the literature refers to the properties of ethanol and does not describe adequately the pharmacology of the beverages consumed. Both metabolites of alcohol and other components of alcoholic beverages possess pharmacologic properties of their own.

Pharmacokinetic Properties of Ethanol

Ethanol is absorbed rather easily across most mucosae, including, most importantly, those of the stomach and small bowel.[1] Absorption can be demonstrated to occur experimentally across the colonic mucosa and slowly from subcutaneous sites of injections. The vapor may be absorbed from (through) the respiratory tract.

Several factors affect the rate of absorption from the stomach and small bowel.[2] Although the precise mechanism is not understood, the absorption of ethanol from the stomach is delayed by the presence of food.[3] A similar effect is seen with beer (probably as a result of its high carbohydrate content). Ethanol is absorbed more rapidly from the small bowel. Foodstuffs have much less effect on the rate of absorption from the small bowel than from the stomach as a result of the vast surface area of the villous mucosa. Patients who have had a gastrectomy may complain that they are intolerant of moderate doses of alcohol since the beverage is delivered as a bolus to the small bowel.[4]

Studies of subjects who are physically fit and have fasted show that the total absorption time for small-to-moderate doses of alcohol is from two to six hours. These studies suggest also that 20% of a usual dose is absorbed from the stomach and 80% from the small bowel.[5] Such studies, however, are poor approximations to the usual setting of alcohol consumption and to the clinical status of the alcoholic.

The concentration of ethanol ingested also can affect the rate of absorption. High concentrations (up to 30%) have complex effects. They induce pylorospasm, which delays absorption. However, such high concentrations (if present in sufficient quantity over as short a time as one or two hours) induce inflammation in the stomach, and absorption of ethanol across an inflamed mucosa is faster than across a normal mucosa. Intermediate concentrations of ethanol in a beverage (15% to 30%) inhibit gastric motility and secretions but do not cause pylorospasm.

Distribution of ethanol is fairly uniform throughout the body,[6] with the volume of distribution being about 0.55 L/kg. Animal studies indicate that central nervous system (CNS) concentrations are very similar to plasma concentrations, although both animal and human studies show that the cerebrospinal fluid concentration after an acute load lags the plasma concentration during both the ascending and the descending phases. Red blood cells generally contain lower concentrations of ethanol than the surrounding plasma for reasons that are not clear. The uniformity of distribution throughout the body makes a single compartment model adequate for most pharmacokinetic studies.

The elimination of ethanol from the plasma is dependent on its metabolism.[2] Less than 5% of a typical ethanol load is excreted unchanged in the urine. If other drugs are present that compete for the same enzymes as ethanol, a greater proportion of the alcohol load will be excreted unchanged in the urine, yet, this does not significantly hasten the overall rate of elimination. A predictable, negligible proportion of a total load is exhaled, since the concentration of ethanol and alveolar air is in equilibrium with that of arterial blood.[7] This forms the basis for the accurate assessment of intoxication by breathalyzer.

Above an ethanol concentration of 20 mg/dL, the elimination curve from plasma is linear with time,[2] with the average rate of elimination being about 10 mL of ethanol per hour. This is roughly equivalent to a glass of wine (100 mL), a glass of sherry (30 to 50 mL), a small measure of liquor (15 to 20 mL), and less than a bottle of beer (200 mL) per hour. This linear decay curve with respect to time (zero-order kinetics) results from saturation of the metabolizing enzymes, that is, the enzymes are catabolizing ethanol at maximal velocity, independent of the ethanol concentration. At low concentrations of ethanol (less than 10 mg/dL), the enzymes are not saturated, and the elimination of these small amounts of ethanol is exponential (first-order kinetics). In this instance, the velocity of the reaction is directly proportional to the alcohol concentration remaining. Zero-order kinetics have the effect of making metabolism of moderate doses of alcohol slower than if first-order kinetics obtained. Because zero-order elimination occurs even with moderate plasma ethanol levels, a driver could be accused correctly of intoxication and have a positive breathalyzer test at 8 am if he had drunk several beers the previous evening, all before midnight.

The peak plasma concentration of ethanol is dependent predominantly on the rate and extent of absorption and is not greatly affected by the rate of metabolism. The very small increases in the rate of metabolism that may occur in the chronic drinker will not have any appreciable effect on the peak plasma concentrations achieved by a standard dose of alcohol (Fig. 4.1).

The principal metabolite of ethanol is acetaldehyde. Of a number of enzyme systems that have been identified in vitro as capable of catalizing this oxida-

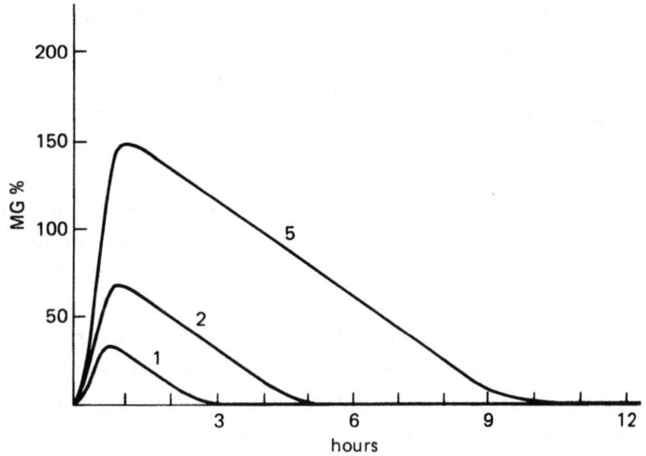

FIGURE 4.1. Typical curves for plasma ethanol concentration following ingestion of one, two, or five drinks.

tion, alcohol dehydrogenase is clearly the most important in vivo.[2] Only a small proportion of ethanol is eliminated by the microsomal enzyme oxidizing system (MEOS). The actions of catalase and a miscellaneous group of enzymes catalyzing glucuronidation and sulfate formation from alcohol have been identified in vitro and in tissues of animal origin, but these reactions are of no practical importance.

Alcohol dehydrogenase is not confined to the liver, and about 10% to 20% of the metabolism of ethanol occurs peripherally. The enzyme, no matter the location, uses nicotine-adenine dinucleotide (NAD) as a cofactor. During oxidation of significant quantities of ethanol, large amounts of NADH are generated, and this change in redox status produces many of the metabolic consequences of alcohol ingestion, as detailed in Part V.

Pharmacodynamic Properties of Ethanol

The pharmacologic, therapeutic, and toxic effects of a drug on the body (ie, what the drug does to the body) are its pharmacodynamics. The effects of ethanol on various organ systems relate to the pathophysiology of those systems.

Central Nervous System

At the cellular level, ethanol is essentially a depressant drug, similar to general anesthetics. However, by preferentially depressing those neurons that are normally inhibitory, an overall stimulatory effect on general behavior occurs when ethanol is used in moderate doses.[6] Because of this effect, alcoholic beverages are widely regarded as stimulants by the layperson. Similarly, interruption of usually inhibitory pathways accounts for the decline in coordination seen with alcohol use, its production of nystagmus, and the initial increase in the vigor of spinal reflexes. Animal experiments indicate that the reticular formation of the brainstem is an especially important site for the depression of inhibitory pathways.

Electroencephalographic (EEG) studies on humans after alcohol consumption show replacement of the alpha-rhythm with a slow rhythm. At equivalent blood ethanol levels, this effect is reported to be less in alcoholics. The clinical significance of these EEG changes is not clear.

Effects on the sensorium are varied. All psychometric measurements of coordination and reaction time are adversely affected by alcohol, even at plasma concentrations well below those legally determined to be the upper limit for driving an automobile. As the plasma ethanol concentration rises, the first higher functions to be impaired are those most dependent on prior experience and learning, such as discretion and social modesty. People with abnormally high (ie, performance-limiting) levels of anxiety can experience beneficial anxiolysis with a small amount of alcohol. At higher plasma concentrations, defects in memory, flights of ideas, and mood swings all appear. Individuals vary significantly with regard to euphoriant and hallucinogenic effects of alcohol, and the responses change according to the type and strength of the alcoholic beverage, the environment in which it is drunk, and the person's previous history of alcohol intake.[8]

In even moderate doses, ethanol is an analgesic in many people.[9] The analgesia produced is similar to that of opiates rather than local anesthetics. It involves distraction from and disinterest in the source of pain rather than reducing awareness of pain or severity of a painful stimulus.

At high doses, ethanol is a nonspecific depressant of the CNS. Reduction in level of consciousness and in the vigor of all reflexes and depression of the vasomotor and respiratory centers may be seen.

Ethanol inhibits the release of antidiuretic hormone (ADH) from the neurohypophysis, resulting in water diuresis.[10] There is no effective diuresis of sodium, however, and ethanol has no therapeutic use as a diuretic.

Peripheral Nervous System

Concentrations of ethanol of 5% to 10% are required to interrupt peripheral nerve conduction effectively. These levels are achieved by local injection, a procedure used to treat chronic pain from a localized source.[6] Interruption of conduction is long term or permanent.

Cardiovascular System

The effects of alcohol on the cardiovascular system (CVS) are complex. At low doses of alcohol, the cardiovascular reflexes remain intact; at high doses, orthostatic hypotension, depression of CVS reflexes, and syncope and its precursors are observed.[11] Cerebral blood flow in the horizontal subject is unaffected until very high concentrations of alcohol have been achieved (about 300 mg/dL), when it is marginally reduced. It is not known if this effect, observed only at poisonous plasma concentrations, is direct or reflects reduced cerebral metabolism in general.

Small vessels (primarily arterioles) are dilated by moderate doses of ethanol. This occurs at plasma concentrations much lower than the concentrations required to produce vasodilation when applied topically, suggesting a central effect. The commonly reported sensation of warmth associated with ingestion of alcoholic beverages can be attributed to this effect in the skin.[11] Cutaneous vasodilation increases the risk of hypothermia in cold climates and may be a cause of rosacea in the alcoholic. Although alcohol is as effective as glyceryl trinitrate in treating angina pectoris in some people, it does not improve accompanying electrocardiographic (ECG) ST segment and T wave changes. There is no evidence that alcohol dilates small vessels in the coronary vasculature or that it increases either myocardial oxygen supply or efficiency.

Gastrointestinal Tract

The acute effects on the gastrointestinal tract are many and varied.[12] The results depend on the state of the organ system before exposure and on the dose, preparation, and timing of the drink. Alcohol in moderate doses produces central stimulation of both salivation and gastric secretion. At higher doses, motility of the stomach is reduced, and there is direct damage to all exposed mucosae.

Libido

Nothing has been written that can outshine the immortal bard, who wrote [*Macbeth* Act 2, Scene 3 (1623 folio)]:

Macduff: What three things doth drink provoke?
Porter: Marry Sir, nose-painting, sleep, and urine.
Lechery, Sir, it provokes, and unprovokes; it provokes the desire, but it takes away the performance.

Modern researchers, using penile plethysmography and vaginal pressure studies, confirm Shakespeare's observations.[13]

With chronic ethanol abuse, testosterone levels fall. This results from the toxic effect of ethanol on the testes, from hyperestrogenism, and from induction of hepatic enzymes, with a resultant increase in the rate of testosterone metabolism.

Mechanisms of Tolerance to Alcohol

Acquired (as opposed to innate) pharmacologic tolerance develops with habitual use of ethanol. Three varieties of acquired tolerance to drugs are recognized: (1) Drug-dispositional tolerance results from changes in the pharmacokinetic properties of the agent and occurs because of increased rate of metabolism, causing reduced concentrations of the drug at its site of action. This variety of tolerance has little effect on the peak intensity of action. (2) Pharmacodynamic tolerance results from adaptive changes within affected systems, and responses are reduced at the same concentrations of the drug. (3) Behavioral tolerance is change resulting from behavioral mechanisms.

It is clear that pharmacodynamic tolerance to ethanol develops. In psychometric testing in both men and animals, chronic exposure to alcohol produces improvement in performance even though plasma concentrations of ethanol are unchanged.[14]

This type of adaptive mechanism is seen with other sedative drugs and has been best studied with the opioids (Fig 4.2). Acutely, the opioids bind to specific receptors on noradrenergic nerve endings (those in the brainstem being most critical). The binding decreases the release of norepinephrine in response to a stimulus, with concomitant diminution of response. With chronic administration of opioid, increased sensitivity of the postsynaptic neuron mediating the response develops so that the lesser amounts of norepinephrine released cause a normal response. Similar changes are seen with chronic administration of ethanol, but the mechanism of these ethanol-induced adaptive changes is unknown. Indeed, there is no evidence that a specific receptor for ethanol exists.

Dispositional changes with chronic ethanol intake occur, but they are quantitatively insignificant with regard to the pharmacokinetics of ethanol, although they are important with regard to some interactions between ethanol and other drugs. Induction of the MEOS occurs in both animals and man, but the elimination of ethanol in chronic drinkers remains zero order and similar to that of the occasional user.

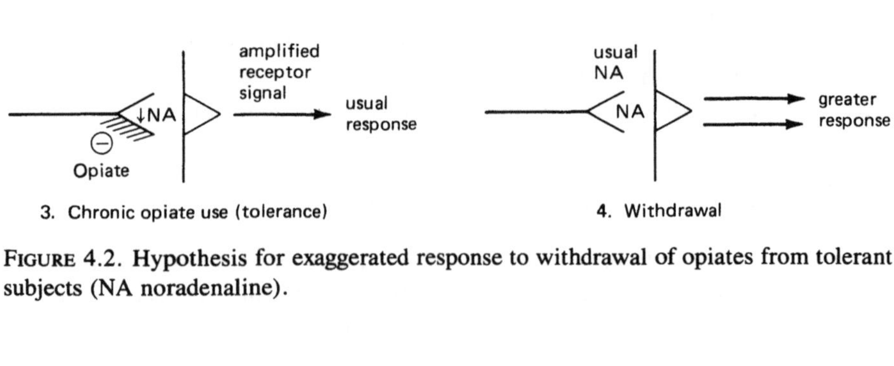

FIGURE 4.2. Hypothesis for exaggerated response to withdrawal of opiates from tolerant subjects (NA noradenaline).

Physical Dependence and the Withdrawal State

Physical dependence on ethanol develops as the result of chronic intake of large amounts of alcoholic beverages. Withdrawal reactions (abstinence syndrome) are the expression of physical dependence and occur when there is a relative decrease in blood ethanol levels. Like those for tolerance, the mechanisms for the development of physical dependence and withdrawal from ethanol have not yet been elucidated. Current evidence suggests that both phenomena are intimately related, are mediated by ethanol itself, and represent the expression of adaptive mechanisms at the subcellular level.[8,14-16] Alcohol withdrawal is not associated with any morphologic changes in the brain, and the syndrome is almost always fully reversible, suggesting a functional or metabolic derangement as the primary etiology. It has been proposed that when ethanol and other depressant drugs (Fig. 4.2) are ingested in large amounts over prolonged periods of time, depressant activity over certain areas of the CNS occurs. In response to this chronic stimulus, these areas undergo adaptive metabolic changes aimed at restoring normal function.[14] These adaptive responses, which are appropriate in the presence of ethanol, become overactive when the depressant is discontinued and are clinically manifested by a state of systemic hyperexcitation, or withdrawal syndrome. When the depressant drug is removed gradually, adaptive responses are reduced and withdrawal is either absent or mild.

There are several hypotheses concerning neurochemical and neurophysiologic mechanisms responsible for physical dependence and the withdrawal syndrome. These include the concept of enzyme induction, in which ethanol inhibits the rate-limiting enzyme in a metabolic pathway leading to the synthesis of a substance, perhaps a neurotransmitter. This inhibition is then followed by a compensatory increase in the synthesis of enzyme and consequent CNS hyperstimulation on withdrawal. Inhibition by alcohol of the synthesis or effects of a neurotransmitter may result in changes at the receptor level, with increases in receptor density or sensitivity. These changes in receptor function then lead to augmentation of neurotransmitter effects when the inhibitory effects of alcohol are removed.

The withdrawal syndrome develops when a period of relative or absolute abstinence decreases ethanol blood levels in a person who is chronically intoxicated. It should be emphasized that even a reduction in the amount of alcohol ingested could precipitate a withdrawal syndrome.[9,17] The severity of the syndrome is proportional to the duration and magnitude of ethanol consumption. Chronic alcoholics usually reduce or stop their drinking involuntarily. The most common causes for abstinence are lack of funds, accidents with injuries requiring hospitalization, and alcohol-related illnesses. Many episodes of alcohol withdrawal occur while the patient is hospitalized, and the physician should be aware of the early clinical manifestations. The major manifestations of alcohol withdrawal are tremulousness, hallucinosis, seizures, and delirium tremens (DTs).

These may occur independent of each other or, more frequently, in various combinations.[8,9,17]

In the early stages of withdrawal and usually after an overnight period of abstinence, the patient complains of nervousness, irritability, and gastrointestinal symptoms, particularly nausea and vomiting. Tremulousness, the most common manifestation of withdrawal, is a prominent feature at this stage, and patients refer to it as "the shakes" or "the jitters." Occasionally, the patient may complain of a "shaky feeling inside" without objective evidence of tremor. The symptoms tend to recur every morning and are quickly relieved with a few drinks. If no ethanol is ingested, the symptoms may worsen, depending on the degree of physical dependence, and reach a peak at 24 to 36 hours. The patient has coarse, generalized tremors, which are fast (6 to 8 cycles/second) and irregular and are exacerbated by motor activity and emotional stress. Other manifestations at this stage are hyperalertness, tendency to startle easily, inattentiveness, insomnia, anorexia, tachycardia, mild disorientation in time, and poor recent memory. The symptoms tend to subside within a period of a few days to one week, although the hyperalertness and feelings of uneasiness may last up to two weeks.[8,9]

Hallucinosis occurs in approximately one quarter of the patients with tremulousness and appears within 24 to 48 hours of abstinence, although the onset may be delayed up to one week. This syndrome lasts from a few days to two weeks; however, a small proportion of patients may develop chronic auditory hallucinations associated with other symptoms characteristic of paranoid schizophrenia.[8,9] The patient complains of nightmares and disturbed sleep, and there is misinterpretation of sounds and shadows, especially in the darkness. The hallucinations can be visual, auditory, or mixed. Very rarely, they are olfactory or tactile. More than 80% are visual; they may be terrifying and are often animate, with representation of human and animal forms. Auditory hallucinations may be in the form of threatening human voices. The response of the patient tends to be appropriate for the content of the hallucination, and suicide and homicide have been reported. After the episode is over, the patient can recall the hallucinations quite vividly and is aware of their unreality.

Grand mal seizures may occur in nonepileptic patients during alcohol withdrawal.[8,9,17] The EEG is normal during the intervals between convulsions. Seizures usually occur within eight to 48 hours after the cessation of drinking and may be in the form of a single seizure or in bursts of two to six or more. Occasionally, a patient will develop delirium tremens, but seizures very rarely follow this entity. The onset of focal seizures should always suggest the presence of a focal lesion, for example, a subdural hematoma secondary to head trauma.

Delirium tremens is the most dramatic and serious manifestation of ethanol withdrawal, occurring in about 4% of all alcoholics admitted to a general hospital.[8] The onset is usually within two to four days after the cessation of drinking, and single episodes rarely last more than 72 hours. Delirium tremens is characterized by a state of severe confusion, agitation, tremulousness, hallucinosis, and signs of markedly increased sympathetic discharge, such as tachycardia, diaphoresis, hypertension, hyperthermia, and dilated pupils. Hypomagnesemia and respiratory alkalosis are commonly associated findings. Very rarely, relapses will occur during a period of four to five weeks after the first episode. After the episode subsides, the patient falls into a profound sleep and awakens lucid and exhausted, without much recollection of what has happened. Mortality rates for DTs vary from 2% to 15% with a decrease in recent years as more attention has been paid to medical complications. Trauma and complicating illnesses, such as aspiration pneumonia, cirrhosis, pancreatitis, and gastrointestinal bleeding, worsen the prognosis significantly. Patients usually die in a state of hyperthermia or peripheral circulatory collapse. Pathologic examination of the brain is unrevealing, and routine laboratory tests fail to show any specific or predictable abnormality.[18,19]

Alcohol as a Therapeutic Agent

The layperson may regard alcohol as a treatment for almost any ill. Distillation was the invention of the Arabs, and when introduced into the Gaelic culture, the liquor was given the name *Usquebaugh*, meaning the water of life. Not only is this the origin of our word "whiskey," but it accurately reflects the many archaic therapeutic uses of ethanol.

There is some evidence that moderate alcohol consumption confers protection against ischemic heart disease (IHD),[20] since high-density lipoproteins (HDL) have been shown to be negatively associated with IHD, and alcohol consumption may be associated with higher serum HDL levels.[21] However, the mechanism for this remains unclear, since alcohol increases the HDL-3 subfraction rather than the antiatherogenic subfraction HDL-2.[22] The apparent protective effect of moderate drinking, which is small ($RR = 0.5$)[21] cannot be connected to alcohol consumption with certainty because of other differences between abstainers and consumers of alcohol.[23,24] It would be imprudent to recommend increased alcohol consumption as a reliable therapeutic maneuver, since the putative effect is marginal and increased alcohol intake could have vast social and medical consequences. Certainly, an increase in HDL is reversed with any degree of alcoholic liver disease.[21]

Ethanol is used as a solvent and vehicle for many otherwise insoluble drugs. It has bactericidal properties and is used as a preservative and on the skin before an invasive procedure. In addition, as many experienced nurses will testify, it is an astringent and can be of assistance in the management of pressure areas for the bedbound. Ethanol may stimulate the appetite, especially in the elderly. Ethanol is useful in intravenous feeding regimens (7 kcal/g) with awkward requirements for calories and restrictions on volume. The use of ethanol for nerve blockade has been discussed previously. Ethanol treatment of poisoning with methanol, ethylene glycol, and isopropanol is described subsequently.

The Pharmacology of Acetaldehyde and of Congeners

Acetaldehyde is the principal first metabolite of ethanol. The first step is rate limiting for the whole metabolic pathway, so the concentration of acetaldehyde in the plasma is constant for any plasma ethanol concentration above 20 mg/dL. Brien and Loomis published a very good review of the pharmacologic effects of acetaldehyde.[24]

At moderate plasma concentrations, acetaldehyde has sympathomimetic effects on the CVS, including both positive chronotropic and inotropic effects on the heart, peripheral vasoconstriction, and activation of the baroreceptor reflexes. Plasma concentrations of this magnitude are most likely to occur in patients taking disulfiram or drugs with disulfiram-like effects. Many of the CVS effects observed in animals can be abolished by pretreatment with reserpine, a drug that depletes stores of norepinephrine.

Acetaldehyde at high concentrations causes liver toxicity. Mitochondria consume less oxygen, gluconeogenesis is inhibited, and glycolysis is stimulated. These effects combine to produce hypoglycemia. None of these effects can be blocked with propranolol, suggesting that it is a direct effect of the molecule rather than an indirect action via the sympathetic nervous system. Acetaldehyde is, in turn, oxidized to acetate by the NAD-dependent enzyme, acetaldehyde dehydrogenase.

Congeners are small molecules other than ethanol in alcoholic beverages. In wine, these are enanthic esters (usually of heptanoic acid and beneficial to the character of the wine), fusel oil (isomers of amyl alcohol and detrimental to the taste), and methyl anthranilate (which smells like orange blossoms and is agreeable to some palates only). In addition to these esthetic molecules, there are varying amounts of acetaldehyde, ethyl acetate, ethyl formate, methanol, propanol, isobutanol, and isoamyl alcohol. Comparing various types of beverage, it is generally true that the presence of all these compounds varies; a beverage with a high concentration of one congener will probably have high concentrations of them all. The scale from highest congener content to lowest is bourbon, brandy, wine, Scotch whiskey, Canadian whiskey, beer, gin, vodka, and ethanol solutions used in research.[25] There is a diuretic principle in juniper oil that is found in most types of gin.

Many of these congeners have been used as industrial solvents and paint strippers, and some of their known pharmacology is derived from studies of occupational toxicity. All of them are irritants to mucosae in their liquid form, and most are also as vapors. All provoke nausea, and at high concentration, all depress the CNS. In studies of normal volunteers after consumption of alcoholic beverages with varying congener content, it was shown that congeners enhance the sedative effects and prolong the nystagmus of alcohol.

Special forms of toxicity are associated with some congeners, although the mechanisms involved are not well understood. For example, ethyl acetate is a hypoglycemic agent. Methanol through its two metabolites, formaldehyde and formate, is toxic to the optic nerve. Methanol is a major component of wood alcohol or methylated spirits and is added in order to make inexpensive alcohol preparations undrinkable. However, some alcoholics are not deterred from drinking such products and report that methanol has a sweetish taste.

Interactions Between Ethanol and Other Drugs

A drug interaction is an effect that results with two drugs but not with either drug alone. Although there are reports of interactions between ethanol and many drugs in clinical use, few of these interactions are clinically significant. The effect of ethanol on other therapeutic agents is more important clinically than is the effect of other agents on ethanol.

Pharmacokinetic Interactions

Absorption

The effects of ethanol on absorption of drugs involves an interplay of several factors. Ethanol may increase absorption by increasing the solubility of a drug, or by causing mucosal inflammation. Decreased absorption due to ethanol-induced pylorospasm is seen for drugs not absorbed from the stomach. However, ethanol-drug interactions at the absorption phase are seldom of clinical importance. For example, the pharmacodynamic interaction between ethanol and a benzodiazepine[26] is of far more clinical relevance than any increase in benzodiazepine absorption that might occur with concomitant ethanol ingestion.

Anticholinergics slow the rate of absorption of ethanol in the small intestine by retarding gastric emptying. Conversely, metoclopramide speeds gastric emptying and hastens ethanol absorption. Drugs that inflame the gastrointestinal tract mucosa, for example, aspirin, are potentiated in this effect by ethanol.[6]

Distribution

Chronic alcoholism is frequently accompanied by hypoalbuminemia, which is most marked in those whose primary source of calories is ethanol. Many drugs are conveyed in the plasma in equilibrium between the free drug in solution and the drug bound to protein, usually albumin. That portion of drug bound to protein is both pharmacologically inactive and protected from excretion or metabolism. It is the free drug that is pharmacologically active. Thus, an interpretation of total plasma levels of certain drugs (eg, phenytoin) in an alcoholic must be made in conjunction with the plasma albumin. A plasma level in the normal range may be excessive, since a greater proportion of the drug assayed is free and pharmacologically active.[27] For phenytoin, this can occur with plasma albumins reduced to only 30 g/L (normal 33 to 35 g/L). The plasma albumin must be less than 20 g/L for furosemide and 10 g/L for digoxin, before this effect is relevant.

Metabolism

Alcohol dehydrogenase is a nonspecific enzyme capable of oxidizing almost any alcohol molecule. It is the site of competition between ethanol and other alcohols. This is of great importance in cases of poisoning by ethylene glycol, methanol, and rarely isopropanol, all of which may be drunk in deliberately self-destructive behavior or, more commonly, as a less expensive way to become intoxicated.[28] Ethylene glycol is converted via its aldehyde to oxalate and methanol to formaldehyde and formate. These metabolites are more toxic than their parent alcohols, since they produce acidosis and specific organ damage—oxalate on the liver and formate on the optic nerve and the liver.

The aim of treatment for these poisonings is to promote the excretion of the unchanged alcohol. By taking advantage of the higher affinity (lower Michaelis constant, K_m) of ethanol for the alcohol dehydrogenase, one can achieve this with infusions of ethanol.[29] The production of acetaldehyde and acetate occurs at the expense of the production of oxalate, formaldehyde, and formate, and the glycol or methanol is excreted unchanged in the urine in larger amounts. Infusions of ethanol to maintain a plasma concentration of about 100 mg/dL are effective.

Chronic alcohol consumption in man is associated with an increase in activity of the MEOS. This can, in turn, enhance the metabolism of other drugs, including barbiturates, isoniazid, phenytoin, morphine, warfarin, and tolbutamide,[6] so that standard doses of these drugs may be less effective in alcoholics. Both acetaminophen (paracetamol) and carbon tetrachloride poisoning are more serious in those with induced MEOS, since their toxicities depend on toxic metabolites generated by MEOS.

The interaction involving acetaldehyde and disulfiram is an important one, and the therapeutic use of this interaction is discussed in Chapter 8. Disulfiram inhibits aldehyde dehydrogenase, producing acetaldehyde levels in the plasma, for a standard alcohol load, of up to 10 times normal.[30] The toxic effects of acetaldehyde at high concentrations are flushing, hypotension, tachycardia, and sensations of malaise. Not all the effects seen when ethanol is ingested by a person taking disulfiram are reproducible by experimental acetaldehyde infusion. Drug-induced alterations of sympathetic nervous system function may contribute to the overall clinical picture.

In certain people, any of a number of drugs in combination with alcohol can produce a disulfiram-like syndrome.[31] Examples include tolbutamide, phentolamine, furazolidine, quinacrine, chloramphenicol, moxalactam antibiotics, griseofulvin, and metronidazole. The mechanisms leading to the syndrome in these interactions are unclear. These drugs are used frequently, and alcohol is ingested often by patients taking these agents, yet the syndrome is only infrequently observed. This suggests an idiosyncratic component to the interaction and raises the possibility that the mechanism is only partially similar to that of disulfiram.

As previously described, congeners compete with ethanol for alcohol dehydrogenase. In addition, animal experiments demonstrate that twice as much pure ethanol is required to produce a standard degree of MEOS induction as ethanol administered in the form of whiskey. This suggests a possible physiologic role for congeners in MEOS induction in humans.

Pharmacodynamic Interactions

Pharmacodynamic interactions[32] between ethanol and other drugs are fewer. All sedatives are supra-additive with ethanol, and cross-tolerance and cross-dependence are seen with benzodiazepines, chloral hydrate, chlormethiazole, barbiturates, and paraldehyde.[33] Although the sedative effects of phenothiazines, opiates, anticholinergics, and antihistamines are also potentiated by ethanol, cross-dependence and cross-tolerance are not seen. The use of glyceryl trinitrate and ethanol is a very hypotensive combination because the former drug dilates large vessels and alcohol dilates the smaller ones. Tyramine is a congener in many alcoholic beverages, including beers and red wines (especially chianti). The hypertensive crisis seen with monamine oxidase inhibitors is well recorded.[34] There is renewed clinical interest in this group of antidepressants, especially in the treatment of phobic conditions, and since the interaction may be life threatening, great care must be exercised by both physicians and patient about the patient's diet.

The actions of the powerful drugs contained in alcoholic beverages are multiple, complicated, and may be seen in both nonaddicted and addicted patients. Ethanol and its congeners can change the actions of other, prescribed drugs. Physicians should keep these complexities in mind when they treat patients who use or abuse alcohol.

References

1. Auty RM, Branch RA: Pharmacokinetics and pharmacodynamics of ethanol, whiskey, and ethanol with isopropyl, isobutyl, and isoamyl alcohols. *Clin Pharmacol Ther* 1977;22:242–249.
2. Hawkins RD, Kalant H: The metabolism of ethanol and its metabolic effects. *Pharmacol Rev* 1972;24:67–157.
3. Welling PG: Pharmacokinetics of alcohol following single low doses to fasted and nonfasted subjects. *J Clin Pharmacol* 1977;17(4):199–206.
4. Broitman S, Gottlieb L, Vitale J: Augmentation of ethanol absorption by mono and disaccharides. *Gastroenterology* 1976;70:1101–1107.
5. Wilkinson PK: Pharmacokinetics of ethanol after oral administration in the fasting state. *J Pharmacokinet Biopharm* 1977;5(3):207–224.
6. Ritchie JM: The aliphatic alcohols, in Goodman AG, Goodman LS, Rall TW, Murad F (eds): *The Pharmacological Basis of Therapeutics*, ed 7. New York, Macmillan, 1986, pp 372–386.
7. Martin E, Moll W, Schmidt P, Dettli I: Pharmacokinetics of alcohol in human breath, venous and arterial blood after oral ingestion. *Eur J Clin Pharmacol* 1984;26:619–626.

8. Schenker S. The effects of alcohol on the brain: clinical features, pathogenesis and treatment, in Lieber CS (ed): *Medical Disorders of Alcoholism. Pathogenesis and Treatment*. Philadelphia, WB Saunders, 1982, Vol 22: *Major Problems in Internal Medicine Series*, pp 480–525.
9. Victor M, Adams RD: The effect of alcohol on the nervous system. *Assoc Res Nerv Ment Dis Res Publ* 1953;32:526–573.
10. Beard JO, Mott DH: The effect of alcohol on fluid and electrolyte metabolism, in Kissin B, Begleiter H (eds): *The Biology of Alcoholism*. New York, Plenum Press, 1971, vol 1, *Biochemistry*, pp 353–375.
11. Wallgren H, Berry H: *Actions of Alcohols*. New York, American Elsevier, 1970, vols 1,2.
12. Burbige EJ, Lewis DR, Halsted CH: Alcohol and the gastrointestinal tract. *Med Clin North Am* 1984;68:77–89.
13. Wilson GT: Alcohol and human sexual behaviour. *Behav Res Ther* 1977;15:239–252.
14. Kalant H, LeBlanc AE, Gibbons RS: Tolerance to and dependence on some non-opiate psychotropic drugs. *Pharmacol Rev* 1971;23:135–191.
15. Goldstein A, Goldstein DB: Enzyme expansion theory of drug tolerance and physical dependence, in Wikler A (ed): *Addictive States*. Assoc Res Nerv Ment Dis Res Publ, Baltimore, Williams & Williams, 1968, pp 265–267.
16. Collier HOJ: A general theory of the genesis of drug dependence by induction of receptors. *Nature (Lond)* 1965;205:181–182.
17. Behnke RH: Recognition and management of alcohol withdrawal syndrome. *Hosp Pract* 1976;11:79–84.
18. Tavel ME, Davidson W, Batterton TD: A critical analysis of mortality associated with delirium tremens. A review of 39 fatalities in a nine-year period. *Am J Med Sci* 1961;242:18–29.
19. Rohan IE: Alcohol and ischaemic heart disease: a review. *Aust NZ J Med* 1984; 14:75–80.
20. Devenyl P, Robinson GM, Roncari DA: Alcohol and high density lipoprotein. *Can Med Assoc J* 1980;981–984.
21. Gonzalez ER: Unresolved issue: Do drinkers have less coronary heart disease? *JAMA* 1979;242:2745–2746.
22. Haskell WL, Camargo C jr, Williams PT, et al: The effect of cessation and resumption of moderate alcohol intake on serum high density lipoprotein subfractions: A controlled study. *N Engl J Med* 1984;310:805–810.
23. Marmot MG: Alcohol and coronary heart disease. *Int J Epidemiol* 1984;12:160–167.
24. Brien JF, Loomis CW: Pharmacology of acetaldehyde. *Can J Physiol Pharmacol* 1983;61:1–22.
25. Murphree HD, Greenburg LA, Carroll RB: Neuropharmacological effects of substances other than ethanol in alcoholic beverages. *Fed Proc* 1967;26(5):1468–1473.
26. Sellers EM: Ethanol-psychotropic drug interactions: Pharmacokinetics. *Psychopharm Bull* 1984;30(3):497–499.
27. Perucca E: Plasma protein binding of phenytoin in health and disease: Relevance to therapeutic drug maintenance. *Drug Monit* 1980;2:331–344.
28. Dreisbach RH: *Handbook of Poisoning*, ed 11. Los Altos, Calif, Lange Medical, 1983.
29. Cooper JR, Kim MM: Biochemical aspects of methanol poisoning. *Biochem Pharmacol* 1962;11:405–416.
30. Kitson TM: The disulfiram-ethanol reaction. *J Stud Alcohol* 1977;38:96–113.

31. Linnoila M, Mattilla MS, Kitchell BS: Drug interactions with alcohol. *Drugs* 1979;18:299–311.
32. Kissin B: Interactions of ethyl alcohol and other drugs, in Kissin B, Begleiter H (eds): *The Biology of Alcoholism*. New York, Plenum Press, 1974, vol 3, *Clinical Pathology*, pp 109–161.
33. Dundee JW, Howard AJ, Isaac M: Alcohol and the benzodiazepines: The interaction between ethanol and chlordiazepoxide and diazepam. *Q J Stud Alcohol* 1971;32: 960–968.
34. Houslay MD, Tipton KF: Multiple forms of monoamine oxidase: Fact and artifact. *Life Sci* 1976;19:467–478.

Part III
Primary Care of the Alcoholic Patient

This section addresses the primary care of the alcoholic patient from the initial visit through the treatment process to long-term follow-up, whether the patient is drinking or sober. The chapters provide a logical, stepwise approach in caring for the alcoholic, with particular attention to handling denial.

Joan Savitsky emphasizes that a careful history is the most effective tool in diagnosing early alcoholism. She points out that familiarity with the landscape of problem drinking is essential because it is the number of symptoms, rather than any specific one, that is most helpful in making a diagnosis. She describes several sets of questions, including the CAGE questionnaire, which are useful in screening for alcoholism and identifies findings in the medical history, physical examination, and laboratory work that may provide clues to the diagnosis of alcoholism.

Once the diagnosis is known, the physician must ensure that the patient receives appropriate treatment. This process begins, according to Henrietta Barnes, with presenting the diagnosis to the patient. She describes particular barriers to discussing a diagnosis of alcoholism and then outlines strategies for dealing with these difficulties. Educating and establishing a working alliance with the patient are crucial because successful treatment requires that the patient make behavioral changes. Methods of handling the patient who denies the diagnosis or refuses therapy are described.

Picking up on this last point, JudyAnn Bigby begins her chapter with specific plans that can help the physician and patient clarify the diagnosis and the need for treatment. Once the patient and physician have agreed on the need, they can establish realistic short-term and long-term goals and decide on appropriate therapy. Dr. Bigby outlines criteria for preferring office treatment alone versus referral to an alcoholism counselor. Different types of outpatient treatment for alcoholism are reviewed. The section on recovery emphasizes that the first weeks of abstinence are a critical period. Dr. Bigby describes the characteristic features of early abstinence, including the prolonged withdrawal syndrome, and the importance of a supportive and involved physician. She then addresses the common problem of relapse and notes some therapeutic responses. The subsequent chapter by Henrietta Barnes reviews the pharmacology of disulfiram and its role as an adjunctive agent in the treatment of alcoholism.

The decision to detoxify an alcoholic patient on an outpatient basis raises issues of patient safety and comfort. Alan Abrams discusses how to evaluate a patient for outpatient versus inpatient detoxification, including medication protocols, and how to use the detoxification period as a means of initiating long-term treatment for alcoholism.

The treatment of the hospitalized alcoholic patient has two components: management of the alcohol withdrawal syndrome and initiation of rehabilitation. Booker Bush outlines current treatment of major withdrawal syndromes, including seizures. He describes the general physician's role as a primary physician and as a medical consultant in ensuring treatment of the primary disease of alcoholism.

5
Early Diagnosis and Screening

JOAN SAVITSKY

In any discussion of early diagnosis and screening, it becomes evident that there is an overlap between the definition of alcoholism, the natural history of the patient, and confrontation leading to treatment. What are we really looking for? If alcoholism is not present now, might it be in five years?

The goal in screening for alcoholism is to understand the individual's relationship to alcohol. Just as it is inadequate to say, "The patient admits to having an occasional chest pain," it is incomplete to describe a patient's drinking as "social" or that he "has an occasional drink." The physician needs to know how the patient uses alcohol (now and in the past), whether there are problems with work, health, friends, or family that may be related to drinking, and what the patient's risk factors for alcoholism are. These data create a rich, detailed picture that allows the physician to address the patient's individual condition. It is more meaningful and more useful to understand where the patient is currently on the spectrum of drinking behavior than whether or not he is alcoholic.

In 1862, Marcet, a physician, made the following observation about a patient's drinking[1]:

> On first applying to his medical advisor, the patient will probably not state the cause of his illness, and thus seriously mislead the physician in his estimation of the nature of the complaint.

It remains a diagnostic challenge to elicit an accurate drinking history from many patients. There is no computerized tomography or nuclear scan to reveal occult alcoholism. Although laboratory work can be suggestive, results may also be entirely normal. For many alcoholics (especially those in the early stages of developing alcoholism or those who binge drink), alcohol has an impact on aspects of their social and professional lives before it has an obvious effect on physiology.

A probing and sensitive history, obtained from an evasive and denying patient, is still the best tool for revealing problem drinking. Information about a person's use of alcohol is obtained both by explicit questioning and by being alert to other clues in the history, physical examination, and laboratory findings. Vaillant points out that trying to decide when an individual moves from moderate social drinking to alcoholism is like trying to decide when yellow becomes green in the color spectrum.[2] This chapter focuses on subtle clues, the constellation of signs and symptoms, that should alert the physician to possible early problems with alcohol. In some cases, a definite answer will not emerge; the picture may seem more yellow than green. However, even if the patient does not meet rigorous criteria for having alcoholism, incipient problems may exist and will benefit from attention. The situation is similar to that of a 40-year-old, overweight man with borderline high blood pressure and blood sugar who will benefit more from intervention at this point than from treatment of the chronic illnesses he will develop ten years later. Applying some of the screening tools that follow should help the doctor and patient decide on the appropriate type of attention: aggressive intervention, early education, or observation over time.

To explore the five aspects of alcohol use that often indicate underlying problem drinking or the potential for a problem, the physician should determine:

Is there loss of control over the use of alcohol?
Is there evidence of addiction or tolerance?
Are there adverse consequences from drinking?
What is the quantity of alcohol consumed?
What are the risk factors for alcoholism?

The process of taking an alcohol history has its own dynamics. Asking a patient with an alcohol problem about his drinking can cause defensiveness and introduce a sense of wariness into the physician–patient relationship. The idea is not to create an adversarial situation in which the diagnosis is made at the patient's expense but rather to elicit gently the necessary information. As the interview progresses, this material is fed back to the patient. Since therapy begins with the patient's recognition of a problem, treatment has begun.

Screening

Screening for alcoholism may occur as a part of the complete history and physical examination or in the more restricted setting of an episodic encounter. Each physician should develop his own series of questions to explore in a succinct but meaningful way the patient's use of alcohol. As part of the initial screening, the CAGE questionnaire or another screening instrument may be used.[3,4] Regardless of which series of questions are used, two points should be emphasized. The first is that screening for alcoholism involves awareness of the larger picture as well as attention to a few specific questions. The patient who is divorced, out of work, and seeking help for abdominal distress needs to be questioned again and again about alcohol use, even if initial screening does not suggest a problem. The second point is that restating questions several times in slightly different forms may yield inconsistencies and evidence of problems related to drinking that were not apparent initially.

Many situations arise in an episodic care setting in which screening for alcoholism may be appropriate. The physician should screen patients with gastrointestinal distress, elevated blood pressure, tachycardia, tremulousness, or nonspecific symptoms such as malaise and anxiety. A physician prescribing an anti-inflammatory agent must ensure that aspirin is not mixed with copious amounts of beer. When the diagnosis of a potential problem with alcohol is an incidental finding, it is appropriate to confront the patient immediately if he is not likely to return for future visits or to recommend a follow-up appointment for further evaluation and care.

The CAGE Questions

The CAGE questions[3] (Table 5.1) were developed as a general screening tool for occult alcoholism. If all the answers are negative, it takes only a few minutes. If one or more responses are positive, further elaboration of the questions can provide the opportunity for thorough exploration of the patient's drinking patterns. Not all physicians will choose to apply the CAGE questions in each encounter, but it is valuable as an easily remembered (and easily taught) approach to elucidating the role of alcohol in a patient's life. The CAGE questions do not deal with quantity but address issues of control, symptoms of addiction, and some of the adverse consequences that can occur when an individual drinks heavily.

1. **C** Have you ever felt you ought to CUT DOWN on your drinking?
   Further information should be obtained by asking for details: When? What was it like? Why did it not work? Also, related to the first question about control: Have you ever planned to limit your drinking, then found you drank more than you intended? These questions explore prior attempts to control drinking. If there have been such attempts at control, they may indicate sufficient repercussions from drinking to stimulate a change in drinking behavior. Efforts to control drinking also convey a sense of struggle around the use of alcohol. The question of control is central to an individual's relation to alcohol. Loss of control is typically intermittent and unpredictable. Vaillant's data show difficulty with control to be reasonably sensitive and specific for underlying alcoholism.[2]
2. **A** Have people ANNOYED you by criticizing your drinking?
   An affirmative response to this question reveals defensiveness on the part of the patient and gives some indication of the impact his drinking has on those around him. Vaillant's data showed that "defining alcohol abuse by complaints of family or friends captured most of the alcohol abusers at the expense of including (some) drinkers who were otherwise problem free."[2] However, the original paper discussing the CAGE questions found that this question yielded far more false-negative answers than did the three other questions.[3]
3. **G** Have you ever felt bad or GUILTY about your drinking?
   A discussion of one or more drinking episodes that led to feelings of guilt will provide information about adverse consequences. Did the patient suffer physi-

TABLE 5.1. CAGE questionnaire.

C	Have you ever felt you ought to CUT DOWN on your drinking?
A	Have people ANNOYED you by criticizing your drinking?
G	Have you ever felt bad or GUILTY about your drinking?
E	Have you ever had a drink first thing in the morning (EYE OPENER) to steady your nerves or get rid of a hangover?

From Ewing J, Mayfield D: CAGE. *Am J Psychiatry* 1974;131:1121–1123. Reprinted with permission.

cally or fail at something because of drinking? Was someone close to him hurt or embarrassed or disappointed?

4. **E** Have you ever had a drink first thing in the morning (EYE OPENER) to steady your nerves or get rid of a hangover?
   The use of alcohol in the morning after drinking implies withdrawal symptoms relieved by further drinking. This is not the same as having a mimosa at Sunday brunch.

Alternative Approach to Screening

The following questions about the use of alcohol can be incorporated into a routine, nonthreatening inquiry about other habits (smoking, drinking coffee).

How often do you use alcohol?
This starts out as a nonjudgmental assumption that the person does use alcohol. It focuses on frequency, which tends to be answered more accurately than a question about the amount of alcohol used.[5]

How much do you usually use?
Responses to this question are often unreliable, since many alcoholics underreport their use of alcohol. Nevertheless, pressing the patient for specific answers can reveal an ongoing struggle around alcohol. For example, an older woman reported she had gotten into the habit of having two glasses of Scotch each night since her husband died. When pressed, she admitted that over time the amount of Scotch in each glass had increased from one to three ounces. This represents a rather transparent attempt to reassure both herself and the physician that she was not developing a problem with her drinking.

Have you ever used alcohol more heavily?
This question may identify the person engaged in a struggle to control drinking or the person apparently drinking asymptomatically who has a past history of serious problems with alcohol.

These three questions determine the quantity of alcohol the patient is now using or has used in the past and enables the physician to place the use of alcohol into one of three categories: (1) so minimal as to cause no concern, (2) moderate, requiring more information, and (3) definitely excessive. A sense of quantity helps the physician anticipate the severity of withdrawal symptoms the patient may experience. Quantity is a much maligned concept in alcohol screening, both because it does not focus on essential information about what happens when the person drinks and because of the possible erroneous information obtained. However, these approaches to quantification can be useful.

It is also important to assess risk for alcoholism:

Does anyone close to you drink heavily?

This will highlight the individual at risk, since alcoholism is a familial disease. For example, a young man comes to the physician for a routine school physical. Although CAGE negative, he drinks two or three beers each night and has had one blackout. His father was alcoholic. This man is not himself alcoholic, yet he uses alcohol regularly and has a significant family history for alcoholism. He would benefit from education about alcohol and deserves close observation over time to monitor for the potential evolution of drinking problems. Asking whether anyone else drinks heavily may also reveal social upheaval in the patient's life caused by a close relationship with someone who is alcoholic. A referral to Al-Anon or to an alcohol counselor may be beneficial.

Red Flags

It is important to watch for "red flags" as the rest of the history unfolds: divorce, difficulty with work, a history of trauma or arrest.[4,5] Each is nonspecific but, with other information, can provide meaningful data about adverse consequences from alcohol use. Similarly, a history of other drug use or abuse is important in the general assessment of any patient as an indicator of substance abuse and sociopathic behavior. It should prompt attention to possible problems with alcohol.

Driving while intoxicated (as opposed to a history of arrest for DWI) does not make a diagnosis of alcoholism but should be discussed in the same spirit of preventive and educational medicine that leads physicians to question patients about the use of seatbelts. A history of DWI is not diagnostic but should clearly alert the doctor to the possibility of problems with alcohol.

The response to the question, "Why don't you drink?" directed at abstainers may elicit information about past difficulty with drinking or a history of parental alcoholism. Also interesting are Vaillant's data that show teetotalers to be less psychologically healthy than modest social drinkers. According to Vaillant[2]:

> . . . abstainers, like the alcohol abusers, were twice as likely to use defenses associated with character disorder, to take tranquilizers, and to have received a psychiatric diagnosis from a clinician.

The physician must note what is unspoken: the quality of the patient's responses. The person for whom alcohol is not a problem will respond in much the same way as to the rest of the interview questions. The occult alcoholic may be defensive, angry, or evasive. He may respond by attempting to convince the physician (and himself) that he does not have a problem by reciting a litany of all the things he does not do: "I never drink alone, I don't drink every day, I never miss work."

Other Questions to Pursue

If concern is raised by preliminary screening questions or by a constellation of red flags, a series of additional questions can be asked while taking a history. These questions are tools that allow further exploration of a patient's drinking behavior.

What are the circumstances in which you drink?
If the patient's social network is built around drinking with friends or if other members of his immediate family are heavy drinkers, abstinence will be that much more difficult. The significance of this fact should not be underestimated. The suggestion that a patient give up alcohol may imply that he must give up his friends and create new social supports for himself. Alcoholics Anonymous (AA) can be useful in this respect. It provides an alcohol-free environment to replace the loss of drinking companions.

Do you like yourself better when you drink?
A positive answer to this question indicates that alcohol may serve a profoundly important function for the individual. For the alcoholic, drinking starts and is recalled as an experience that is enjoyable and positive. The physician should be aware of this aspect of alcoholism as he attempts to help a patient give up alcohol.

Do you use alcohol as medication to relieve pain, anxiety, or trouble sleeping?
Such use of alcohol may imply significant psychologic or physiologic dependence on alcohol.

Have you had blackouts?
This does not refer to loss of consciousness but, rather, to loss of memory for events while intoxicated. The drinker may behave normally as observed by those around him, but the next day he will have no recollection of what occurred. Surprisingly, blackouts occur relatively early in the evolution of problem drinking and may contribute to denial.

Is your drinking different now than it was five years ago?
The answer to this question may provide insight into a previous or evolving problem with alcohol. It may also reveal a change in tolerance, either increased or decreased over the years. If the patient tells the physician he used to drink hard liquor but now drinks only beer or he used to drink every day but now only drinks on weekends, he may be trying to convince the physician and himself that no problem exists.

Trauma Scale[4]
This scale (Table 5.2) may be particularly useful in an emergency room setting where the prevalence of alcohol-related injury is high.

TABLE 5.2. Trauma scale.

Since your eighteenth birthday
Have you had any fractures or dislocations to your bones or joints?
Have you been injured in a road traffic accident?
Have you injured your head?
Have you been injured in an assault or fight (excluding injuries during sports)?
Have you been injured after drinking?
The score is computed by the number of positive responses (0–5). A score of 2 or more is suggestive of the presence of excessive drinking or alcohol abuse.

Adapted from Skinner HA, Holt S, Schuller R, et al: Identification of alcohol abuse using laboratory tests and a history of trauma. *Ann Intern Med* 1984;101:847–851. Reprinted with permission.

Michigan alcoholism screening test (MAST)[6]

The CAGE questions are drawn from this list of 25 questions designed to screen for occult alcoholism (Table 5.3). Most physicians find it too long and cumbersome to apply in a routine interview. It is included here to provide some idea of other questions that have been associated with problem drinking and because it is referred to in the literature on alcohol.

Many questions used commonly in alcohol screening were designed for and tested on white, middle-aged, male alcoholics. This does not exclude their use in other situations, but the constellation of problems may be difficult. This is especially true in the elderly, where a small amount of alcohol can cause problems that may be attributed incorrectly to the effects of aging. Such special populations are discussed in Part VI.

Problems and Physical Complaints Related to Alcohol

A variety of complaints are associated with alcohol excess:

Gastrointestinal symptoms

- Morning retching, nausea, vomiting, anorexia[7]
- History of gastritis[7–9] or nonspecific acid-peptic distress[7]
- Symptoms of gastroesophageal reflux—alcohol causes decreased lower esophageal pressure and interference with esophageal peristalsis[7]
- Recurrent diarrhea—Alcohol can increase the rate of transit in the small bowel by decreasing impeding peristaltic waves without affecting propulsive movement[7–10]
- Gastrointestinal disturbances that are relieved by alcohol may be caused by alcohol withdrawal

Palpitations[10–12]

Sleep disturbance, anxiety, depression[7,8]

"Nonspecificitis"—multiple somatic complaints with emotional overlay may originate in the distress of excessive drinking

TABLE 5.3. Michigan alcoholism screening test (MAST) questionnaire.

Question	Points
1. Do you feel you are a normal drinker?	2
2. Have you ever awakened the morning after some drinking the night before and found that you could not remember a part of the evening before?	2
3. Does your spouse (or parents) ever worry or complain about your drinking?	1
4. Can you stop drinking without a struggle after one or two drinks?	2
5. Do you ever feel bad about your drinking?	1
6. Do friends or relatives think you are a normal drinker?	2
7. Do you ever try to limit your drinking to certain times of the day or to certain places?	0
8. Are you always able to stop drinking when you want to?	2
9. Have you ever attended a meeting of Alcoholics Anonymous (AA)?	5
10. Have you gotten into fights when drinking?	1
11. Has drinking ever created problems with you and your spouse?	2
12. Has your spouse (or other family member) ever gone to anyone for help about your drinking?	2
13. Have you ever lost friends or girlfriends or boyfriends because of drinking?	2
14. Have you ever gotten into trouble at work because of drinking?	2
15. Have you ever lost a job because of drinking?	2
16. Have you ever neglected your obligations, your family, or your work for two or more days in a row because you were drinking?	2
17. Do you ever drink before noon?	1
18. Have you ever been told you have liver trouble? Cirrhosis?	2
19. Have you ever had delirium tremens (DTs), severe shaking, heard voices, or seen things that were not there after heavy drinking?	2
20. Have you ever gone to anyone for help about your drinking?	5
21. Have you ever been in a hospital because of drinking?	5
22. Have you ever been a patient in a psychiatric hospital or on a psychiatric ward of a general hospital where drinking was part of the problem?	2
23. Have you ever been seen at a psychiatric or mental health clinic or gone to a doctor, social worker, or clergyman for help with an emotional problem in which drinking played a part?	2
24. Have you ever been arrested, even for a few hours, because of drunk behavior?	2
25. Have you ever been arrested for drunk driving or driving after drinking?	2

Score points for negative answers to questions 1, 4, 6, and 8 and positive answers to all other questions. A score of 5 or more points is indicative of alcoholism.

From Seltzer ML: The Michigan alcoholism screening test: The quest for a new diagnostic instrument. *Am J Psychiatry* 1971;127:89–94. Reprinted with permission.

Clues on the Physical Examination

The following findings may be the earliest physical signs of alcohol abuse. They do not include the multiple and dramatic abnormalities seen in the later-stage alcoholic.

Alcohol on the breath or, alternatively, an overwhelming odor of mouthwash
Tremulousness
Tachycardia
Hypertension[13-16]

The physician should rule out occult alcoholism in the hypertensive patient, especially the young hypertensive male. Further work is needed to clarify the effect of alcohol on blood pressure during acute intoxication, in the withdrawal phase, and chronically. No mechanism for the hypertension has been established. It may be corticosteroid excess, action through the renin–angiotensin system, or increased catecholamine synthesis.[14,15]

Clues in the Laboratory

Results of various laboratory tests may indicate alcohol abuse.

Blood alcohol level (BAL)

A level of over 150 mg/dL without gross evidence of intoxication implies tolerance to alcohol and meets NCA criteria for the diagnosis of alcoholism.[17]

Gamma glutamyl transferase (GGT)

This enzyme is induced by heavy alcohol intake over several weeks. Unlike the transaminases, ALT and AST, it does not signal hepatic damage. It usually returns to normal over a period of weeks to months.[18] Various investigators have concluded that the GGT level correlates significantly[19–21] or not at all[18] with the quantity of alcohol consumed. In addition, it is not specific for alcohol use; the GGT may be elevated in both acute and chronic liver disease unrelated to alcohol, as well as with certain drugs, such as phenobarbital and dilantin. In spite of these limitations, the GGT level can be useful as a piece of supplementary data in the context of other information about the patient's alcohol history.

Aspartate aminotransferase (AST, SGOT), alanine aminotransferase (ALT,SGPT)[7]

These may be elevated in fatty liver, as well as alcoholic hepatitis, cirrhosis, and nonalcoholic liver disease. The AST may be greater than the ALT in alcoholic hepatitis and cirrhosis because alcohol has a direct inhibitory effect on ALT synthesis.

Red blood cell indices[22,23]

Elevated mean corpuscular volume (MCV) can result from a direct effect of alcohol on the marrow, as well as from alcohol's effect on folate metabolism. It may be seen also in nonalcoholic liver disease. The MCV may remain elevated after three months of hospitalization. Therefore, it is not a very useful test to follow drinking over the short run.

Elevated uric acid

The metabolism of alcohol produces lactic acid, which competes with uric acid excretion at the level of the kidney.[24]

Discussion

Screening for alcoholism is a process that occurs in all phases of the physician–patient encounter. Formal screening tools have been developed to facilitate this process. From these formal instruments, physicians should evolve their own repertoire of questions that can be asked quickly and expeditiously, serving as a basis for a more detailed history, if appropriate. More important than which specific questions are used is familiarity with the landscape of problem drinking. When signposts to problems occur, the physician must be able to recognize and pursue them.

Studies have attempted to assess how various questions—with or without laboratory work—correlate with a diagnosis of alcoholism. Although such studies help to clarify the utility of different screening modalities, they are subject to exactly the pitfall we try to avoid, that is, they form conclusions about the effectiveness of a test or instrument based on some independent gold standard. In fact, there is no real gold standard for alcoholism in the sense of one test that is ideally sensitive to, and specific for, the problem. In addition, the model used in these studies creates two categories: alcoholic and nonalcoholic. These models are relatively insensitive indicators of problem drinking and miss the incipient alcoholic whose drinking deserves attention.

The MAST was tested against a validation score derived by searching records of every medical facility and social agency in Washtenaw County, Michigan, and reviewing records of the county probation department and arrest records and traffic violations from the state police.[6] Although this provided thorough and objective information, it failed to identify those people whose problems had not yet come to institutional attention.

Screening techniques face a difficulty inherent in any testing process: determining the existence of a problem without including people falsely diagnosed. A study of the CAGE questionnaire showed that there were no false positives among those who responded to all four questions affirmatively. Of all the patients designated alcoholic (based on information collected from different sources), 57% were included among those responding positively to two, three, or four questions. Another way of looking at this is that 43% of the alcoholics escaped diagnosis by this criterion. Of those misidentified by the CAGE questionnaire, either as false positive or false negative, a substantial proportion in the group were psychotic.[3] Subsequent reviews of the CAGE questions indicate sensitivities between 72% and 91% and specificities between 77% and 96% for patients hospitalized on general medical, surgical or psychiatric wards.[19,21,25]

The MAST questionnaire was applied to a variety of different groups (five in all), including hospitalized alcoholics and drivers arrested for DWI. Of the hospitalized alcoholics, 98% scored over five points (considered a positive test). Slightly more than half of those arrested for DWI and drunk-and-disorderly conduct scored in this range. Among 15 subjects who scored in the nonalcoholic range and were subsequently found to be alcoholic by other means, there were many falsities and omissions in response to the MAST questions.[6] It is interesting to note that both in this group and in the CAGE group, false negatives were often attributed to either psychotic or intentionally manipulative behavior. This observation reinforces the importance of attention to all aspects of the patient's presentation.

In one evaluation of the MAST, the questionnaire was given to 99 hospitalized alcoholics with explicit instructions to lie about their drinking. The results were that "despite these instructions . . . no less than 92 percent disclosed sufficient information for them to be classified as alcoholics." This is a vivid demonstration of how important information can emerge in spite of denial.[6]

Mayfield and Johnston applied a series of interview and laboratory techniques in an attempt to determine the most effective screen. They noted that although the biologic tests were more specific than the questionnaires, they were both less sensitive and less efficient in revealing alcoholism.[21] This is not surprising, since adverse social consequences may occur before any physiologic effect in an early alcoholic or binge drinker. They then combined each laboratory value with each questionnaire and found that the particular combination of the BAL with the MAST provided the greatest increase in sensitivity with no loss of specificity. This may be useful in some people, but the long list of questions that form the MAST does not lend itself to a spontaneous and conversational exploration of drinking. The BAL is reasonably expensive and may be negative in early alcoholism or binge drinking. For these reasons, this combination is probably more relevant to research than to clinical practice and is not useful for preliminary screening. As an initial approach, it is preferable to use the CAGE questions (or other questions specifically about the use of alcohol) with attention to the rest of the history, the physical examination, and the routine laboratory work.

Alcoholism in its earliest stages is an insidious, private process marked by denial of its consequences. The physician's attempt to understand a patient's alcohol use often involves surmounting obstacles and persisting in data collection. Synthesizing the data obtained in all aspects of the encounter paints a picture more compelling than any one of its components. In real life, it may take time—a number of visits or even months—to paint a recognizable picture.

No one test, question, or series of questions has been shown to be absolutely specific for and sensitive to occult alcoholism. However, attention to the cumulative effects of drinking can provide an understanding of its role in the patient's life. According to Vaillant, ". . . it was the number of alcohol-related problems, not any particular cluster, which best predicted alcoholism."[2]

References

1. Marcet W: *On Chronic Alcoholic Intoxication: With an Inquiry on the Influence of the Abuse of Alcohol as a Predisposing Cause of Disease, ed 2.* London, John Churchill, 1862. As quoted in: Skinner HA, Holt S, Israel Y: Early identification of alcohol abuse: 1. Critical issues and psychosocial indicators for a composite index. *Can Med Assoc J* 1981;124:1141–1150.
2. Vaillant GE: *The Natural History of Alcoholism: Causes, Patterns, and Paths to Recovery.* Cambridge, Mass, Harvard Univ Press, 1983.
3. Mayfield D, McLeod G, Hall P: The CAGE questionnaire: Validation of a new alcoholism screening instrument. *Am J Psychiatry* 1974;131:1121–1123.
4. Skinner HA, Holt S, Schuller R, et al: Identification of alcohol abuse using laboratory tests and a history of trauma. *Ann Intern Med* 1984;101:847–851.
5. Skinner HA, Holt S, Israel Y: Early identification of alcohol abuse. 1. Critical issues and psychosocial indicators for a composite index. *Can Med Assoc J* 1981;124: 1141–1150.

6. Selzer ML: The Michigan alcoholism screening test: The quest for a new diagnostic instrument. *Am J Psychiatry* 1971;127:89–94.
7. Holt S, Skinner HA, Israel Y: Early identification of alcohol abuse. 2. Clinical and laboratory indicators. *Can Med Assoc J* 1981;124:1279–1294.
8. Eckardt M, Hartford T, Kaelber C, et al: Health hazards associated with alcohol consumption. *JAMA* 1981;246:648–666.
9. Geokas M, Lieber C, French S, Halsted C: Ethanol, the liver, and the gastrointestinal tract. *Ann Intern Med* 1981;95:198–211.
10. West LJ, Maxwell DS, Noble EP, Solomon DH: Alcoholism. *Ann Intern Med* 1984;100:405–416.
11. Singer K, Lundberg WB: Ventricular arrhythmias associated with the ingestion of alcohol. *Ann Intern Med* 1972;77:247–248.
12. Ettinger PO, Wu CF, DeLa Cruz C, et al: Arrhythmias and the "holiday heart": Alcohol-associated cardiac rhythm disorders. *Am Heart J* 1978;95:555–562.
13. Klatsky AL, Friedman GD, Siegelaub AB, Gérard MJ: Alcohol consumption and blood pressure. Kaiser-Permanente Multiphasic health examination data. *N Engl J Med* 1977;296:1194–1200.
14. Saunders JB, Beevers DG, Paton A: Alcohol-induced hypertension. *Lancet* 1981; 1:653–656.
15. Potter JF, Beevers DG: Pressor effect of alcohol in hypertension. *Lancet* 1984; 1:119–122.
16. Clark LT: Alcohol use and hypertension. *Post grad Med* 1984;75:273–276.
17. Criteria Committee, National Council on Alcoholism: Criteria for the diagnosis of alcoholism. *Ann Intern Med* 1972;77:249–258.
18. Robinson D, Monk C, Bailey A: The relationship between serum gamma-glutamyl transpeptidase level and reported alcohol consumption in healthy men. *J Stud Alcohol* 1979;40:896–901.
19. Bernadt MW, Mumford J, Taylor C, et al: Comparison of questionnaire and laboratory tests in the detection of excessive drinking and alcoholism. *Lancet* 1982;2:325–328.
20. Sanchez-Craig M, Annis H: Gamma-glutamyl transpeptidase and high-density lipoproteins cholesterol in male problem drinkers: Advantages of a composite index for predicting alcohol consumption. *Alcohol Clin Exp Res* 1981;5:540–544.
21. Mayfield DG, Johnston RGM: Screening techniques and prevalence estimation in alcoholism, in Fann WE, Karacan I, Pokorny AD, Williams RL (eds): *Phenomenology and Treatment of Alcoholism*. New York, Spectrum Publications, Inc., 1980.
22. Shaw S: Biological markers for the diagnosis of heavy drinking. *Prac Gastroenterol* 1983;7:20–25.
23. Wu A, Chanarin I, Levi AJ: Macrocytosis of chronic alcoholism. *Lancet* 1974; 1:829–831.
24. Lieber CS, Jones DP, Losowsky MS, Davidson CS: Interrelation of uric acid and ethanol metabolism in man. *J Clin Invest* 1962;41:1863–1870.
25. Ewing JA: Detecting alcoholism: The CAGE questionnaire. *JAMA* 1984;252: 1905–1907.

6
Presenting the Diagnosis: Working with Denial

HENRIETTA N. BARNES

Many physicians feel uncomfortable about discussing a diagnosis of alcoholism with a patient. The goal is straightforward enough: the patient must understand that his drinking is a problem and that treatment is necessary. Yet, the patient's denial of the problem or refusal to consider treatment can thwart even the best-intentioned efforts. An understanding, systematic approach to denial can help the newly diagnosed patient begin to engage in treatment, although he may require multiple confrontations over time before accepting the need for treatment. Repeated discussions with no immediate results may frustrate the physician, but the cumulative effect can disrupt the pattern of alcoholic drinking. Many recovered alcoholics state anecdotally that such an encounter "ruined" their enjoyment of drinking, even though their behavior did not change for some time.[1]

The boundaries of this chapter are somewhat arbitrary because the process of diagnosing the disease, presenting the findings to the patient, and negotiating appropriate treatment often overlap. Successful intervention requires the physician to gather data, counter denial, and provide hopeful support simultaneously.

Obstacles to Presenting the Diagnosis

Discussing the diagnosis of alcoholism with a patient is never easy. The patient's denial, the relapsing nature of the disease, and the negative attitudes and experience of the physician all conspire against open and fruitful interchange. Awareness of these different factors enables the physician to address each obstacle explicitly.

The major barrier to discussing the diagnosis of alcoholism is the patient's denial. By realizing that denial is primarily the result of unconscious psychologic mechanisms (no matter how willful it may appear), the physician can maintain a sympathetic, therapeutic stance despite an angry, denying patient. Generally, the rigidity of a patient's denial parallels the severity of the disease and the depth of his fear and shame.[2] Attempts to present the diagnosis may be met with rationalizations about drinking behavior or attempts to minimize the amount or its consequences:

You'd drink, too, if you had four young kids at home and your husband was on the road most of the week.

I don't know why the cops stopped me for drunk driving. I'd only had a couple, and there was hardly a dent on the other car.

An obvious contradiction of the facts may represent severe denial, such as when a late-stage alcoholic living on the street described himself: "I may be a bum, but I'm not an alcoholic."[2]

A vague and inconsistent history is often a clue to underlying alcoholism and suggests organic impairment. Repeated intoxication, blackouts, and chronic memory deficits result in distorted recollection of past events:

A Hispanic woman who denied any alcohol intake gave a history of multiple surgical procedures, but she could not remember when they were performed or in what hospital. Her physician attributed the vague history to lack of education and her inability to speak English until she appeared in the emergency unit in alcohol withdrawal.

Cognitive deficits are also problematic in presenting the diagnosis. The patient may not remember the discussion or may selectively recall only the least threatening aspects of it:

One week after a lengthy discussion of his alcoholism with his physician, a severely alcoholic patient could remember only that "three or four drinks might be affecting his blood pressure."

Disagreements with family members who accompany the patient to an appointment are another expression of denial. Although family members can help the patient hear the diagnosis, the physician must be aware that families often participate in the alcoholic's denial.[3] The Griners discuss the complicated dynamics of denial within an alcoholic family in Chapter 19.

The diagnosis of alcoholism carries many negative implications. At best, acceptance of the diagnosis implies a long-term commitment to abstinence, a terrifying prospect to the alcohol-dependent person. For the physician, it means continued attention to a chronic, relapsing condition with serious medical, psychologic, and social sequelae, or it means the responsibility for making an effective referral. At worst, alcoholism connotes hopelessness and moral turpitude, attributes that only confirm the alcoholic's low self-esteem. If the physician shares these beliefs, there is little incentive to confront the problems of alcoholism.[4,5]

Physicians may have other difficulties in discussing alcoholism with patients. Inadequate training, specifically lack of supervised clinical experience treating alcoholism, limits a physician's effectiveness.[6] Concerns about the normalcy of the physician's own drinking may make the physician reluctant to discuss a patient's alcoholism,[7] especially if the patient is from a similar socioeconomic background.[8]

A more thorny problem is the risk of losing a patient after presenting the diagnosis. Even in the hands of a skillful and supportive physician, confrontation is uncomfortable, and many physicians are unfamiliar with this role. One must remember that confrontation, although painful, is not harmful,[9,10] and avoiding a discussion of the diagnosis of alcoholism only allows the patient to continue the cycle of drinking and denial. The physician must weigh the relationship with the patient against the need for explicit discussion.

Strategies for Presenting the Diagnosis

The provocative nature of denial demands a careful response in order to maintain a positive interaction with the patient. The physician can adapt many of the techniques developed for caring for chronically ill or challenging patients[11] to the interview with the alcoholic.

Use Explicit Information

The patient needs to understand concretely how alcohol has interfered with his life. Presenting specific facts from the history, physical examination, or laboratory data that demonstrate the adverse effects of drinking produces better results than a general statement about drinking too much. (The patient will always be able to tell you about a friend who drinks twice as much and has no problems.) Generalizations or hypotheses that the physician cannot support by data are easily refuted by the patient.

Even if the physician thinks that additional information is needed to confirm the diagnosis, it is helpful to share concerns about the patient's drinking problem at whatever level of certainty the data support:

> Your trouble sleeping, your high blood pressure, and your recent problem on the job make me wonder if alcohol may be your main difficulty. We'll need to discuss this further when I see you again.

Be Empathic and Hopeful

Presenting the diagnosis as an expression of concern for the patient's health or safety can further the physician's alliance with the patient. The physician needs to counter the alcoholic's low self-esteem and expectation of rejection by providing a clear message of hope for improvement with treatment. Often an alcoholic's sense of hopelessness is so pervasive that it may envelop the physician. Even when it may seem unwarranted by the history, a posture of therapeutic optimism may interrupt a cycle of drinking and despair. A characteristic and understandable reaction to an alcoholic's denial is to moralize and frighten the patient with threats of dire consequences if drinking continues. However, these negative attitudes only reinforce the alcoholic's hopelessness and are usually counterproductive.

Acknowledging the positive aspects of drinking will reassure the patient that the physician understands how important alcohol is in the alcoholic's life. In order to design an appropriate treatment program, the physician should know what the patient feels he will be losing by becoming sober. The patient who describes alcohol as "his best friend" will need help developing new relationships; one who uses alcohol to slow his racing thoughts may need an evaluation for bipolar depression. By using the analogy of alcohol as a medication with good effects and side effects, the physician and patient can discuss alternatives to alcohol that have fewer negative effects. Sometimes generating a balance sheet of the pros and cons of drinking can help the patient clarify the role that alcohol plays in his life.

Educate about Alcoholism

Many drinkers are ignorant of the basic facts about alcohol and alcoholism, such as the effects of alcohol as a drug, risk factors for developing alcoholism, or signs of early withdrawal. Educating the patient is a nonthreatening way to help him recognize symptoms of alcoholism that may be present.

A discussion of alcoholism as a disease legitimizes seeking medical care for alcoholism per se and not just for its medical consequences. The comparison of alcoholism to other chronic diseases, such as diabetes or hypertension, whose treatment requires behavioral changes reinforces the fact that abstinence from alcohol is therapy and not punishment.[12] Understanding alcoholism as a disease and not as an expression of personal inadequacy or lack of will power allows the patient to identify with the healthier aspects of his personality and address the alcoholism with less guilt.

Avoid Arguments about a Diagnostic Label

Although recovery from alcoholism is predicated on acceptance of the diagnosis, a patient's refusal to call himself alcoholic need not stand in the way of treatment as long as the patient is able to connect his drinking with its negative consequences.[12] Many patients need to deny the diagnosis even while exploring treatment options. Furthermore, the patient's definition of alcoholism may differ from the physician's. It is always useful to know what the patient's conception of the word "alcoholic" is, so that educational efforts can address the patient's specific concerns.

Be Realistic about Your Role and the Patient's Response

Very few alcoholics achieve sobriety on the first attempt, and most will suffer at least one relapse in the process of recovery.[13] Realistic expectations based on an understanding of the disease can prevent the frustration and disappointment that lead physicians and patients to view the problem as hopeless. Rather than accepting denial at face value, the physician can use the apparent contradictions between the facts and the patient's responses as additional data to explore with the patient. For example,

You came to see me about your stomach pain and trouble sleeping. Yet when I suggested that you stop drinking for a while to see if alcohol were causing some of the difficulty, you said drinking had never been a problem for you and there was no reason to stop. Knowing how concerned you are about your health, I wonder why you seem reluctant to stop. Maybe we could talk about what it would be like for you not to drink.

Different clinical situations demand different responses. One-time interactions, such as walk-in or emergency unit visits, are the appropriate setting for explicit confrontation about a person's use of alcohol. There is no long-term relationship to jeopardize, and the patient should receive an unequivocal message that alcoholism is the problem and that recovery is possible.

In working with an intoxicated patient, the physician must keep in mind that the patient is incapable of assimilating information. The interaction should be brief and the recommendations simple[14]:

You've been drinking. Before we can talk about any other problems, you need to get the alcohol out of your system. I can arrange for you to go to detox.

Patient Responses to Hearing the Diagnosis

Mr Jones, a computer salesman, came to the emergency unit because of a flare-up in his shoulder bursitis. Because he was tachycardic and hypertensive, the physician questioned him about his alcohol use. The patient stated he drank "a few beers" at night and gave positive answers to three of the four CAGE questions. When the physician expressed concern that alcohol might be a problem, Mr Jones agreed and said he had not been sure how to get help.

Ms Green, a 30-year-old social worker, acknowledged that alcohol might have played a role in her recent divorce and subsequent depression. However, she said that she "knew all about alcoholism" from her professional work and would take care of the problem herself.

Mr Williams, a real estate broker, had seen several physicians for anxiety, epigastric distress, and hypertension. Because his business involved frequent entertaining, he prided himself on being able to drink heavily with his clients and not become intoxicated. He attributed his symptoms to stress at work and dismissed the idea that alcohol might be involved.

These three vignettes represent patients' characteristic responses to hearing the diagnosis of alcoholism. Each reaction shows a different level of denial and necessitates a different response from the physician.

Patient Agrees to the Problem and Desires Help

Despite the patient's acceptance of the diagnosis, denial is usually present. It may resurface as an unwillingness to discuss in detail problems resulting from the use of alcohol or reluctance to accept specific recommendations for treatment. Many patients expect that they will be able to return to social drinking if they control their drinking in the short run. Although the severity of the disease may preclude a future of social drinking, it could be detrimental for the physician to insist initially that the patient commit himself to lifelong abstinence. The prospect of a life without alcohol may be so frightening to an alcoholic that he will avoid treatment.

Patient Acknowledges a Problem but Refuses Help

By reinforcing the patient's understanding that a problem exists, the physician can begin to develop a therapeutic alliance. The patient needs to perceive discussion about what he will do on his own as concerned inquiry and not rejection. Useful questions include:

How does the current plan differ from previous (presumably unsuccessful) attempts to control drinking?
What will have to happen for the patient to feel he needs outside help?
What is different about this attempt at sobriety?

The physician can be supportive of the patient's efforts even while negotiating with the patient to accept more formal treatment in the event that his plan fails. If the patient is reluctant to agree, the physician must reassess the patient's understanding of the problem and his commitment to changing his drinking behavior.

Patient Denies a Problem with Alcohol

After a careful presentation of the diagnosis, this response may be extremely frustrating for the physician because it appears to preclude further dialogue. Rather than insist that the patient does have a problem, the physician might engage in a discussion of what would constitute a problem with alcohol. Given the usually progressive nature of the disease, the patient may very likely fulfill his own criteria in time.

Respectful acknowledgment of the patient's opinions about his diagnosis may allow the patient to explore further whether alcohol might be a problem. Additional social or family history can be revealing. The patient may agree to participate in an experiment of short-term abstinence or controlled drinking. Additional strategies are outlined in Chapter 7.

Understanding denial is crucial in discussing the diagnosis of alcoholism with an alcoholic patient. Regardless of immediate outcome, presenting the diagnosis of alcoholism can have therapeutic benefits. By raising the contradictions inherent in continuing to drink in spite of known damaging consequences, the physician may help disrupt the pattern of alcoholic drinking. By providing respect, hope, and encouragement, the physician can support the patient's efforts at recovery.

References

1. Cutler DF: Personal communication, 1983.
2. Bean MH: Denial and the psychological complications of alcoholism, in Bean MH, Zinberg NE (eds): *Dynamic Approaches to the Understanding of Alcoholism*. New York, Free Press, 1981, pp 55–96.
3. Paredes A: Denial, deceptive maneuvers, and consistency in the behavior of alcoholics. *Ann NY Acad Sci* 1973;233:23–31.
4. Baekeland F, Lundwall LK: Engaging the alcoholic in treatment and keeping him there, in Kissin B, Begleiter H (eds): *Treatment and rehabilitation of the chronic alcoholic*. New York, Plenum Press, 1977, pp 161–195.
5. Bissel L: Diagnosis and recognition, in Gitlow SE, Peyser HS (eds): *Alcoholism: A Practical Treatment Guide*. New York, Grune & Stratton, 1980, pp 23–45.
6. Warburg MM, Cleary PD, Rohman M, et al: Diagnosis and management of alcoholism: A survey of medical residents. *J Med Educ* (In press).
7. Clark WD: Alcoholism: Blocks to diagnosis and treatment. *Am J Med* 1981;71: 275-286.
8. Wolf I, Chafetz M: Social factors in diagnosis of alcoholism in social and non-social situations. *Q J Stud Alcohol* 1965;26(1):72–79.
9. DiCicco L, Unterberger H, Mack JE: Confronting denial: An alcoholism intervention strategy. *Psychiatr Annals* 1978;8:596-606.
10. Hertzman M: Getting alcoholics out of your office, into treatment, and back into your office. *Primary Care* 1979;6(2):403–416.
11. Groves JE: Taking care of the hateful patient. *N Engl J Med* 1978;8:596–606.
12. Block MA: Motivating the alcoholic patient, in Gitlow SE, Peyser HS (eds): *Alcoholism: A Practical Treatment Guide*. New York, Grune & Stratton, 1980, pp 47–71.
13. Vaillant GE: *The Natural History of Alcoholism: Causes, Patterns, and Paths to Recovery*. Cambridge, Mass, Harvard University Press, 1983.
14. Clark WD: Emergency care of the patient with alcoholism, in Kravis T, Warner C (eds): *Emergency Medicine: A Comprehensive Review*. Rockville, Md, Aspen Systems Press, 1983, pp 517-531.

7 Negotiating Treatment and Monitoring Recovery

JUDYANN BIGBY

For many physicians, the most difficult aspect of treating alcoholic patients is lack of knowledge about what resources are available once the diagnosis is made. Presenting the diagnosis and working with the patient's denial, as discussed in Chapter 6, are the first steps. However, the majority of patients require additional, specific treatment. With adequate knowledge and skills, the primary care physician is in a unique position to take advantage of his special relationship with the patient to facilitate such treatment.

Denial of Diagnosis and Refusal of Treatment

In general, patients who do not acknowledge their problem with alcohol will not agree to participate in a treatment plan, and those who accept the diagnosis will many times refuse specific treatment. For some of these patients, refusal of specific treatment reflects uncertainty about the diagnosis or discomfort in accepting it fully. To help the patient understand the underlying problem and to accept the need for treatment, the following strategies may be used: a trial of controlled drinking, a trial AA meeting, or family intervention.

A two-to-three-week trial of drinking a specified amount of alcohol mutually agreed on by the physician and patient may demonstrate loss of control. The physician must make it clear to the patient that, during the trial, there will be no exceptions to the amount agreed on and that the patient will begin treatment if unable to adhere to the contract. At the end of the trial, if the patient is drinking in a controlled manner, he should be followed closely. If he fails the trial, the lack of control clearly demonstrates the need for treatment. Before the trial begins, the physician should discuss how the patient feels about limiting his drinking to get a sense of the patient's preoccupation with alcohol. If the patient refuses to participate in the trial, the implications should be discussed. The following case illustrates the usefulness of this trial:

A 29-year-old male, referred for evaluation of hypertension, acknowledges drinking large amounts of alcohol daily, including during lunch hour. Further history indicates that alcohol is interfering with his work performance and his relationship with his wife. The patient denies a problem but agrees to drink no more than four drinks per day for a three-week period so that the effect on his hypertension can be assessed. He returns in three weeks, aware that he was unable to limit his drinking. He is then more receptive to the idea that he has a problem and agrees to see a counselor who specializes in alcoholism.

Another intervention that may prove useful is a trial AA meeting, which allows the patient to observe recovered alcoholics who do not fit a stereotypical picture. These are important observations for the patient to make to dispel feelings of hopelessness and to overcome discomfort with the label "alcoholic." The physician should suggest that the patient attend the meeting for educational purposes, rather than as treatment, and assist the patient in choosing a meeting where he will meet people from a background similar to his own. Responses to experiences at meetings vary but are often negative. The patient may be more willing to admit he has a problem but be skeptical about the effectiveness of AA or be unable to deal with the uncomfortable feeling he experiences as he identifies with someone like himself at the meeting.[1] The physician should acknowledge the feelings generated by attendance at AA and encourage the patient to continue with treatment as a means of dispelling some of the pain and discomfort.

An alternate strategy to a trial of controlled drinking or AA meetings is family intervention.[2] Family members or other significant people in the patient's life are interviewed by a counselor specializing in alcoholism (or someone with similar experience) in the patient's absence and urged to describe the adverse effects of alcohol use on each family member personally. Following this, the family, patient, and counselor meet, and individual family members—beginning with the least involved member—recount the facts in a manner that expresses their concern and caring. In most cases, the patient will consent to treatment at this point. Physicians without experience with this technique should not attempt a formal intervention, but nonjudgmental confrontations can be used by the physician in the office. This approach to patients is addressed more fully in Chapter 19.

If the patient continues to deny his alcoholism, he may benefit from a referral to an expert in alcoholism. The physician should make it clear to the patient how the referral may clarify the problem with alcohol. If the denial continues, the primary care physician's responsibility is to follow the patient, emphasizing alcoholism as a major problem, and offering treatment when the patient is most vulnerable and most apt to accept it. The physician should continue to point out discrepancies between attempts at abstinence and stated beliefs that "I could stop drinking any time."[3]

Acceptance of Diagnosis and Agreement to Treatment

The first step in treatment is for the physician and patient to establish short-term and long-term goals. Although the physician and patient may not agree on all the goals, the physician can use the discussion of goals to reinforce the reasons not to drink and ways this can be accomplished. In the long run, it is the patient's responsibility to decide for himself how much of a problem he has and what he will do about it. Short-term goals may include detoxification, treatment of medical problems, education and support of the family, short-term abstinence, and learning new behavior. It is important to discuss this last goal with the patient to enable him to find alternatives to the psychologic defense mechanisms he has been using to deal with uncomfortable feelings.

The long-term goals are to restore self-esteem and heal the medical and social damage resulting from alcoholism. For most patients, these goals can best be achieved by abstinence. It is often unwise to discuss the need for long-term abstinence early in treatment, but it should be discussed as the period of sobriety increases. Although studies describing the natural history of alcoholism show that approximately 5% to 10% of alcoholics may be able to resume social drinking without adverse consequences,[4,5] it is impossible to predict who can and who cannot. Furthermore, it is unclear from the studies what percentage of patients who appear to be normal social drinkers at short-term follow-up will resume alcoholic drinking later.[6] Therefore, it is prudent to encourage total abstinence as the long-term goal.

Referring the Patient for Treatment

The primary care physician should be familiar with local treatment sources and have a contact in the field of alcoholism for formal and informal consultations. The decision to refer the patient to specific agencies depends on the availability of various treatment modalities. Success rates for achieving abstinence are similar for all treatment modalities, including inpatient and outpatient.[7] Such factors as age, sex, ethnic background, and addiction to other drugs are important in determining the appropriate treatment agency. Not all psychiatrists, social service agencies, or mental health agencies can provide treatment for alcoholism, and treatment that does not focus on alcoholism as the primary problem may delay recovery.[8]

The decision whether or not to refer a patient for treatment of alcoholism depends on the physician's interest, skills, and experience and on the resources available in the community. It is often appropriate for the primary care physician to treat the patient suffering from alcoholism in the office while the patient attends AA meetings. Patients who do not want to be referred may leave the physician with no other alternative, and many alcoholics do well with this form of treatment.[7,9] The physician's role is to monitor recovery and offer support, with the help of AA. Physicians who recommend this form of treatment should be familiar with the organization and philosophy of AA, the stages of recovery, and signs of relapse.

Referral of patients to specific alcohol treatment programs is appropriate when the physician feels uncomfortable treating the patient or when it is clear that the patient will need multiple supports in order to achieve and maintain abstinence.

When deciding where to refer a patient, the physician should know the patient's previous treatment experience, his attitude regarding prior treatment, precipitants of relapse, and what treatments the patient felt were most helpful in the past. Patients with multiple attempts at abstinence may require several strategies to maintain abstinence. Families of alcoholics are often unable to accept the diagnosis and, if they are not involved in the treatment plan, may interfere with the patient's attempt at recovery. Family members or significant others may, therefore, benefit from referral to Al-Anon or family therapy.

The following cases illustrate the differences between patients suitable for treatment by the primary care physician and those for whom referral to a more structured treatment program is preferred.

A 55-year-old policeman seeks medical care for leg pain. When asked about his use of alcohol, the patient states that he drinks only beer but for the past two months has abstained because of stomach problems and complaints from his wife that he drinks too much. When he is questioned further, it becomes clear that the patient and several family members are alcoholics. The patient has never had formal treatment for his alcoholism, but one relative who has been abstinent for several years has offered to take him to AA meetings. The patient has gone "on the wagon" several times in the past, remaining sober for two to three months before resuming drinking.

The physician discusses alcohol as a drug and its effect on the body. The patient's own account of the adverse effects of alcohol on his life is used to illustrate the negative effects of drinking. Clearly there is a need to establish a treatment plan for a longer period of abstinence than he has experienced in the past. The physician suggests he go to an AA meeting with his brother before the next visit. Over several months, the patient finds an AA group and a sponsor and remains sober while he continues to see his primary care physician.

A 39-year-old secretary comes for a routine physical examination. She has been hospitalized several times for alcoholic ketoacidosis. She has attended several AA meetings over the past five years, had been hospitalized in an alcohol treatment unit once, and has taken disulfiram briefly. Her longest period of sobriety is three months. She is currently drinking. The patient agrees that she has a problem with alcohol but is angry about not being able to drink as other people do. Previously, her goal had been to reverse the medical complications and then attempt social drinking.

She is referred to an alcohol counselor who arranges for her to attend an AA group for women from similar socioeconomic backgrounds, and she is enrolled in an outpatient alcohol-treatment program. The primary care physician maintains his relationship with the patient and continues to monitor her during the initial stages of recovery, emphasizing the adverse effects of alcohol on all aspects of her life, not just the medical complications.

Outpatient treatment may include some combination of individual, group, or family therapy, often in conjunction with AA, with most private insurance covering this type of service. For patients without insurance, sliding-scale fees may be available. Physicians should consider inpatient therapy if (1) the patient has medical or psychiatric problems requiring close observation, (2) the patient has failed outpatient therapy, or (3) there is an impending psychosocial emergency, such as threat of divorce or job loss. Halfway houses are available in some communities for people without a stable social life who may require a maximum amount of structure to maintain sobriety after detoxification.

Once the physician and patient have established a treatment plan, it is important that the physician discuss the plans and goals with the treatment agency. In most cases, referrals should be made immediately—as soon as the patient agrees—either from the doctor's office or while the patient is hospitalized. The physician should continue to follow the patient during initial treatment and be sure that appointments with counselors are kept and attendance at AA meetings is maintained.

Some alcoholic patients continue to drink despite attempts to intervene by health care providers. These represent the group of alcoholics with the most extreme denial and lowest self-esteem. Most physicians have experienced the frustration and anger associated with caring for these patients, but it is important for physicians to continue to offer treatment periodically, especially at those times when the patient is experiencing the most distress from drinking. Patients who are frequently inebriated can be disruptive, and in order to provide care for them, physicians should set limits defining acceptable behavior while recognizing their own limitations in dealing with such patients.

Recovery

In the early stages of recovery, patients need to establish a relationship with someone who can provide structure and guidance through the physical and psychologic changes that occur. Patients are most vulnerable to relapse during the first six months of sobriety when they are still experiencing physiologic effects from chronic excessive use of alcohol. It is helpful for the primary care physician to continue to see the patient in recovery while the relationship develops between the patient and the counselor, AA sponsor, or therapist.

Acute withdrawal symptoms usually subside in three to seven days, but a large number of patients experience the prolonged withdrawal syndrome. Symptoms may last as long as two years but generally resolve spontaneously in six to 12 months. Symptoms include excessive anxiety, sleep disturbance, sexual dysfunction, depression, emotional lability, and craving for alcohol.[10] After assessing patients for any underlying medical conditions that might cause these symptoms, the physician should reassure the patient that, as abstinence continues, these symptoms will abate. The use of benzodiazapenes or other psychotropic medications should be avoided, since their use may prolong the withdrawal process and may result in dual addiction. It is difficult to assess the appropriateness of antidepressants during the early recovery period, but the symptoms can resolve spontaneously. Typically, recovery is a prolonged experience and may take as long as five years to complete.[11]

Other behavioral problems encountered during the recovery period are euphoria and the dry-drunk syndrome. Patients feel better after a period of abstinence and will often go through a period of euphoria, known as the "pink cloud" in AA jargon, which occurs usually within the first six weeks to two months into recovery. Patients may have the impression that all their problems have been resolved by not drinking. Several months later when psychosocial problems may persist, patients become depressed and are at risk for relapse. Patients with dry–drunk syndrome are abstinent but have not changed their attitudes or behavior regarding the adverse effects of drinking. Typically, the patient with the dry–drunk syndrome complains about not being able to drink, attributes his need for abstinence to some external factor, or continues to deny the real need for abstinence. These patients are at high risk for relapse, have often stopped drinking on their own, and refuse specific treatment.

For the physician, the main tasks during recovery are (1) to establish a treatment plan that protects the patient from relapsing and (2) to help the patient deal with the consequences of previous alcohol abuse and subsequent abstinence. For the patient, the main task during recovery is to learn new ways of reacting to stress, depression, and guilt. It is important to keep reiterating why drinking must stop. As patients recover from the physiologic effects of alcohol on the CNS, they are better able to understand why drinking is harmful, but in the meantime, the physician should emphasize that the desire for alcohol and impulse to drink will diminish over time. The physician should be certain that the patient has worked out a clear plan for dealing with the impulse to drink, for example, has obtained a sponsor in AA. The potential for relapse must be anticipated and discussed.[11]

Patients' feelings during the period of recovery need be acknowledged. They become more acutely aware of missed relationships, lack of success in job or social status, or ill health. In addition, problems attributed to alcoholism may not be resolved totally, and the patient may feel deceived about the need for abstinence. Family members may be angry about the suffering, neglect, and abuse they have experienced or may be unwilling to give up roles they have assumed during the patient's drinking.

Signs of impending relapse include hopelessness, anger, somatic complaints, increasing requests for anti-anxiety medications, and discontinuing treatment. The physician should discuss the implications of these symptoms with the patient. Recommendations should include intensifying the treatment plan, such as increasing the number of AA meetings, obtaining a sponsor, adding an individual counselor, or perhaps inpatient therapy.

The following case illustrates some of the problems encountered during recovery.

The 55-year-old policeman described previously continues to complain of anxiety and sleep disturbance after seven months of abstinence. He has decreased the number of AA meetings he attends and is upset that he continues to crave alcohol and feels irritable and angry.

After acknowledging the distress the patient is experiencing, the physician reassures him that these feelings will not last forever. He is reminded that his relationship with his family has improved and his gastrointestinal complaints have resolved completely. The physician expresses his concern about the patient's symptoms and makes suggestions for increasing treatment, such as attending additional AA meetings and talking with the sponsor, and an appointment is made with a counselor.

Because relapse is common, it should be anticipated. The physician should make it clear that his relationship with the patient will not depend on sobriety and that he is willing to continue treating the patient should relapse occur. If there is a relapse, the physician should explore the precipitants. The patient may have been testing his ability to drink in a normal manner or may have resumed drinking in an attempt to treat the uncomfortable feelings experienced during recovery. The physician should congratulate the patient for the period of abstinence that was achieved and be optimistic about the potential for successful treatment. Previous treatment modalities can be reinstituted with increased supports.

If the primary care physician is aware of the physiologic and behavioral problems associated with early abstinence and relapse, he can help alcoholic patients establish realistic treatment plans and provide knowledgeable support throughout the course of the illness.

References

1. Bean MH: Denial and the psychological complications of alcoholism, in Bean MH, Zinberg NE (eds): *Dynamic Approaches to the Understanding of Alcoholism*. New York, Free Press, 1981, pp 55–96.
2. Johnson V: *I'll Quit Tomorrow*. New York, Harper and Row, 1973.
3. Miller W: Motivational interviewing in problem drinkers. *Behav Psychother* 1983;11:147–172.
4. Vaillant G: *The Natural History of Alcoholism: Causes, Patterns, and Paths to Recovery*. Cambridge, Mass, Harvard University Press, 1983.
5. Vaillant G: The natural history of alcoholism. IV. Paths to recovery. *Arch Gen Psychiatry* 1982;39:127–133.
6. Pendry ML, Maltzman IM, West LJ: Controlled drinking by alcoholics: New findings and a reevaluation of a major affirmative study. *Science* 1982;217:169–175.
7. Emrick CD: A review of psychologically oriented treatment of alcoholism. II. The relative effectiveness of different treatment approaches and the effectiveness of treatment versus no treatment. *J Stud Alcohol* 1975;36:88–108.
8. Vaillant G: Dangers of psychotherapy in the treatment of alcoholism, in Bean MH, Zinberg NE (eds): *Dynamic Approaches to the Understanding of Alcoholism*. New York, Free Press, 1981, p 36.
9. Edwards G, Orford J: A plain treatment for alcoholism. *Proc Roy Soc Med* 1977; 70:344–348.
10. Kissin B: The role of physical dependence and brain damage in the protracted alcohol abstinence syndrome. *Adv Alcoholism* 1981;2(11):1–3.
11. Bean MH: A psychoanalyst's guide to therapy with the problem drinker. (Unpublished)

8
The Use of Disulfiram

HENRIETTA N. BARNES

Disulfiram is a drug commonly used as a deterrent to drinking because of the unpleasant physiologic responses it induces in the presence of alcohol. It has a definite, albeit limited, role in the treatment of alcoholic patients. Several hundred thousand abstinent patients take the drug daily to help overcome the impulse to drink alcohol.[1]

Pharmacology

Disulfiram is an anti-oxidant, first used medically as a scabicide and anthelmintic.[2] Disulfiram inhibits several enzyme systems, most notably aldehyde dehydrogenase and dopamine-β-hydroxylase. The drug is absorbed rapidly but takes 12 hours to be effective because of its tendency to accumulate in fat stores. Elimination is slow; one week after ingestion 20% of the drug is still in the body.[3] Most of the drug is metabolized in the liver and excreted in the urine. Reactions with alcohol can occur five to seven days and have been reported as long as 14 days after the last dose of disulfiram.[4]

Alcohol-Disulfiram Interaction

Fifteen minutes after a person taking disulfiram ingests alcohol, a characteristic syndrome occurs, starting with cutaneous flushing and a feeling of warmth. Subsequently, headache, nausea, vomiting, difficulty breathing, precordial chest pain, hypotension, and syncope may occur.[5] ECG changes of ST depression, T-wave flattening, and QT prolongation are common.[6] Occasionally very severe reactions are reported, including myocardial infarction, seizures, congestive heart failure, and arrhythmias.[2] Fatalities are usually associated with high doses of disulfiram (more than 500 mg daily), the ingestion of more than two drinks of alcohol, or the concomitant use of other vasoactive or psychoactive medications.[7]

The reaction usually lasts about 30 to 60 minutes but may last several hours. A delayed reaction may occur 48 hours after ingesting alcohol. As little as 15 ml of

50% alcohol cough syrup can cause a reaction.[8] Rubbing alcohol, mouthwash, and fumes from alcohol solvents in poorly ventilated areas have been implicated in causing reactions. Because of the possibility of severe reaction, disulfiram may be contraindicated in patients with coronary artery disease, seizure disorders, hypothyroidism, cirrhosis, and nephritis. Patients taking alpha-blockers or beta-blockers or psychotropic medications, such as monoamine oxidase inhibitors, are also at increased risk for a severe hypotensive reaction because these agents block the body's normal compensatory hemodynamic mechanisms.[7]

Treatment of a reaction is supportive, including oxygen, fluids, pressors, and monitoring for cardiac arrhythmias. There is no known specific antidote, although prostaglandin inhibitors and H_2 blockers may decrease the flushing reaction.[7]

Adverse Effects

Initially, most patients experience fatigue and sedation. Mild gastrointestinal disturbances, a metallic or garliclike taste, and an elevated serum cholesterol (responsive to pyridoxine) are common.[9] Generally, reduction in dosage eliminates these annoying effects.

Less common effects include skin rash (5% to 10%), impotence, and mildly abnormal liver function tests. CNS effects include depression and psychosis in susceptible individuals, polyneuropathy, optic neuritis, and acute organic brain syndrome.[10] Disulfiram may produce fetal limb abnormalities if taken by pregnant women.[11]

Interactions with Other Drugs

Disulfiram and paraldehyde produce an interaction similar to disulfiram and alcohol. By inhibiting metabolism, disulfiram increases serum levels of warfarin and phenytoin. Disulfiram interacts additively with isoniazid to produce increased CNS effects, including ataxia and psychosis. Many drugs produce a disulfiram-like reaction if alcohol is ingested. Commonly used drugs producing this reaction include the oral hypoglycemic agents (chlorpropamide, tolbutamide), antibiotics (sulfonamides, chloramphenicol, quinacrine, metronidazole), some nonsteroidal anti-inflammatory drugs (phenylbutazone, phenacetin), ethacrynic acid, and trinitroglycerin.[2,4,12] Disulfiram also delays the metabolism of caffeine, so that patients taking disulfiram who are heavy coffee drinkers may experience nervousness, palpitations, and difficulty sleeping.[13]

Indications in Outpatient Practice

Disulfiram is effective only in the context of ongoing treatment for alcoholism, whether in an alcoholism clinic or with a general physician. A positive relationship with the caregiver is essential. Historically, the use of disulfiram as coercive treatment or adversive conditioning often had negative consequences.[2] In this therapeutic model, disulfiram was viewed psychologically as punishment. Patients were given a loading dose of disulfiram and then challenged with alcohol in order to precipitate a reaction. Initially, fear of the reaction made patients and physicians reluctant to use the drug. As physicians became more experienced with the drug, they understood that disulfiram could be useful as a positive symbol—as a good object replacing the harmful object, alcohol, or as an extension of the therapeutic relationship.[14]

The symbolic use of disulfiram underscores the need for a cooperative patient and education about drug effects. The patient must be willing to take disulfiram and must be fully aware of the consequences of drinking while taking the drug. No patient should be given disulfiram without his full knowledge and understanding. Patients need to know that, unlike other medications sometimes prescribed for alcoholism, disulfiram does not give a high and is not a cure. Full medical and psychosocial evaluations are important before starting disulfiram. Patients who tend to do well on disulfiram are older, well-motivated people with long drinking histories and stable social situations.[15] A patient who has previously drunk while taking disulfiram or who drinks so impulsively that he is not aware of picking up that first drink is a poor candidate for the drug.

Duration of treatment is highly individualized. Some people use disulfiram only in the early months of sobriety, whereas others continue to use it for years or take it on an as-needed basis during periods of stress. Most patients should be followed monthly while taking the medication.

Therapy with disulfiram offers several advantages:

1. The decision not to drink has to be made only once a day. Freed from the preoccupation with drinking, the alcoholic patient is able to participate more productively in other forms of treatment.[16]
2. An impulse to drink must be deferred at least five to seven days, during which time the patient may rethink his decision to drink.
3. Taking disulfiram is a concrete expression of the patient's desire to remain abstinent. Any change in behavior, such as missing doses, is usually the first obvious warning that he is leading up to a drink.

Alcoholic patients may object to taking disulfiram because they see it as a crutch and want to get sober on their own. For patients with previous unsuccessful attempts at sobriety, this stance usually represents a form of denial; the patient is reserving the right to drink. Newly diagnosed patients may require more drinking experiences to prove to themselves that they need help. The analogy of insulin for the diabetic or diuretics for the hypertensive may help the patient accept treatment with disulfiram. It is useful to stress that, even with disulfiram, the patient is responsible for his sobriety because it is he who must take the medication each day.

There is controversy about the use of disulfiram. Critics argue that the dangers of disulfiram outweigh the advantages and that the therapy is based on fear of the alcohol-disulfiram reaction, which is a poor source of motivation. Although AA has no official position on the use of disulfiram, some AA members believe that no drug should be used in recovery and that people taking disulfiram may be dry, that is, not drinking but not working toward a healthy life without alcohol.

Evaluations of disulfiram's efficacy provide conflicting data. A small study in one therapist's practice on the use of disulfiram as an adjunct to counseling showed a longer time to relapse when the patient used disulfiram.[17] However, in a recent Veterans Administration cooperative study, patients treated with disulfiram and counseling did not differ from control subjects, treated with placebo and counseling, in total abstinence, time to first drink, or measures of social stability.[18] Despite the availability of counseling, it is not clear that use of disulfiram was an explicit therapeutic issue.

Dosage and Cost

The usual dosage is 250 mg/day taken at bedtime because of the drug's sedative effects. If side effects occur, the dosage may be reduced to 125 mg/day. The cost of a month's supply of disulfiram is approximately $10.

References

1. Fried R: Comments on Antabuse therapy in alcoholism (Letter). *Alcoholism* 1977;1:275.
2. Kwentus J, Major LF: Disulfiram in the treatment of alcoholism. *J Stud Alcohol* 1979;40:428–446.
3. Ritchie JM: The aliphatic alcohols, in Goodman LS, Gilman A (eds): *The Pharmacological Basis of Therapeutics*, ed 5. New York, Macmillan, 1975, pp 148–149.
4. Editors: Disulfiram (Antabuse). *Medical Letter.* New Rochelle, NY, 1980;22(1):1.
5. Child GP, Osinski W, Bennett RE, Davidoff E: Therapeutic results and clinical manifestations following the use of tetraethylthiuram disulfide (Antabuse). *Am J Psychiatry* 1951;107:774–780.
6. McCabe ES, Wilson WW: Dangerous cardiac effects of tetraethylthiuram disulfide (Antabuse) therapy in alcoholism. *Arch Intern Med* 1954;94:259–263.
7. Sellars EM, Naranjo CA, Peachey JE: Drugs to decrease alcohol consumption. *N Engl J Med* 1981;305:1255–1261.
8. Petroni NC, Cardoni AA: Alcohol content of liquid medicinals. *Clin Toxicol* 1979;14:407–432.
9. Major LF, Goyer PF: Effects of disulfiram and pyridoxine on serum cholesterol. *Ann Intern Med* 1978;88:53–56.
10. Reisberg B: Catatonia associated with disulfiram therapy. *J Nerv Ment Dis* 1978; 166:607–609.
11. Nora AH, Blu J: Limb-reduction anomalies in infants born to disulfiram-treated alcoholic mothers (Letter). *Lancet* 1977;2:664.
12. Seixas FA: Alcohol and its drug interactions. *Ann Intern Med* 1975;83:86–92.
13. Beach CA, Mays DC, Guiter RC, et al: Inhibition of elimination of caffeine by disulfiram in normal subjects and recovering alcoholics. *Clin Pharmacol Ther* 1986;39: 265–270.

14. Wallerstein RS: Psychologic factors in chronic alcoholism. *Ann Intern Med* 1958;48:114–122.
15. Lundwall L, Baekeland F: Disulfiram treatment of alcoholism: A review. *J Nerv Ment Dis* 1971;153:381–394.
16. Weisman MN: The use of disulfiram in the treatment of alcoholism. *Md State Med J* 1968;17:83–84.
17. Fuller RK, Williford WO: Life-table analysis of abstinence in a study evaluating the efficacy of disulfiram. *Alcoholism* 1980;4:298–301.
18. Fuller RK, Branchey L, Brightwell DR, et al: Disulfiram treatment of alcoholism: a Veteran's Administration cooperative study. *JAMA* 1986;250(11):1449–1455.

9
Outpatient Treatment of Withdrawal

ALAN ABRAMS

This book emphasizes the early recognition of drinking problems, yet, physicians often first make the diagnosis of alcoholism only when the patient demonstrates signs and symptoms of alcohol withdrawal. The treatment for withdrawal is only one aspect of the treatment for alcoholism. The office management of the symptoms of acute withdrawal sets the stage for long-term management of the alcoholic patient. Physical dependence on alcohol and the spectrum of withdrawal syndromes are discussed in Chapter 4.

Mr G is a 45-year-old, married office worker in a large firm. He has seen his internist for an annual physical examination for several years. On a routine visit, he complains of several weeks of epigastric pain on an empty stomach. As in previous years, his answers to the CAGE questions are negative, and he states that he only drinks "a few beers" at night, none during the day. On this visit, Mr G is nervous but in no real distress. His blood pressure is 160/100, pulse 90. He has mild epigastric discomfort on abdominal examination, with a guaiac-negative stool. Laboratory results show a normal blood count with a slightly increased mean corpuscular volume. Liver function tests are within normal limits, but an amylase is one and one-half times normal. The presumptive diagnosis is alcohol withdrawal.

Assuming that Mr G is prepared to attempt to stop drinking, how can he be detoxified safely? Should he go home or be admitted?

The physician contacts Mrs G, who agrees to come with her husband for his next appointment in two days to discuss a treatment plan. When they return, Mr G's symptoms are unchanged. He complains of poor appetite. On examination he is mildly shaky but not confused. His blood pressure is still 160/90, pulse 110. Social history reveals that Mr G previously was divorced and remarried. Mrs G does not drink and has been attending Al-Anon meetings for the past six months.

Factors in Deciding to Treat as Outpatient

Mr G's case illustrates those factors a physician must consider in planning detoxification on an outpatient basis (Table 9.1).

TABLE 9.1. Criteria for outpatient treatment of withdrawal.

1. Minor withdrawal symptoms only.
2. Absence of other significant illnesses, including head trauma.
3. Availability of physician or other caregiver daily during withdrawal period.
4. Commitment to complete abstinence from alcohol.
5. Adequate social support network (family or friends).
6. Pre-existing relationship between patient and physician.

Minor Withdrawal Symptoms

The recent history or prior experience with the patient should assure the physician that there will not be complications. Patients who have had delirium tremens or withdrawal seizures are likely to have severe reactions again. Patients with hallucinosis, global confusion, or the appearance of new psychiatric disorders, such as paranoia or seizures, should be admitted for observation.[1]

Mr G appears nervous but with a clear sensorium. The clinician learns from the patient's wife that Mr G has stopped drinking on his own at home previously. At such times, he usually sleeps poorly and seems nervous for two to three days. There has never been any disorientation or seizures. Mr G tells his physician he has not "broken out" as heavily or for as long this time. The physician thus learns that this drinking episode is not as severe as at times in the past. All indicators suggest a smooth, medically uncomplicated, minor withdrawal.

Absence of Other Illnesses

Patients must be free of other medical illnesses that require hospitalization. A thorough history, physical examination, and appropriate laboratory tests should precede the decision to treat the patient at home. Patients should have no history of recent major injuries, especially head trauma. Patients should be well hydrated and reasonably well nournished, although short-term, mild nutritional deficiencies (folate deficiency) do not preclude ambulatory treatment of withdrawal. There should be no evidence of decompensated liver disease or cardiovascular instability. The physician must exclude clinically significant fever (an oral temperature of greater than 38.3°C) and gastrointestinal bleeding. Mental status testing must reveal a clear-thinking individual.[2]

Although Mr G complains of continued epigastric distress and lack of appetite, physical examination does not demonstrate an acute abdomen. Laboratory examination verifies normal electrolytes, liver function, and hematologic parameters. A mild elevation in amylase is of concern clinically, but in the absence of evidence of serious pancreatic, biliary tract, or ulcer disease, the clinical picture appears medically safe at this juncture for ambulatory treatment and follow-up. Both the patient and his wife confirm the absence of spells or major trauma recently.

Availability of Physician

The physician or his designee (nurse practitioner, alcohol counselor) must be able to see the patient for three to five consecutive days to monitor treatment. This close follow-up provides a number of benefits in addition to observing the safety and efficacy of the outpatient detoxification regimen. First, it reaffirms the concept that alcoholism is a serious illness requiring medical attention. Second, it helps establish a positive relationship for the patient who feels isolated and alone. The patient's opportunity to explore a relationship with the physician, so vital to the long-term recovery process, begins with the physician's implicit statement, "I need to see you because I care about how things go for you."[3]

Although Mr G's withdrawal symptoms are mild, the physician asks him to return daily during the withdrawal process to assess his abdominal pains, elevated amylase level, hydration status, and overall clinical course. This close monitoring reassures Mr G and his wife, as well as the clinician.

Patient's Abstinence

The patient must agree to abstain from drinking. Although many patients say that they will cut back or only take a drink if they feel shaky, the physician must require abstinence. The combination of two sedative hypnotics (the pharmacologic agent used for detoxification and alcohol) is risky in an environment without medical supervision. Patients who refuse to abstain are ambivalent about the definition of their problem or desire for treatment. The patient's clear commitment to abstinence allows the physician to offer relief of symptoms through pharmacologic intervention during early withdrawal. When the patient is stable, the clinician must follow up on the commitment to abstinence by encouraging the patient to participate in other support programs. When the goal of abstinence is agreed to early, it increases the patient's compliance and probability of prolonged sobriety.

Availability of Social Supports

The patient must have adequate, reliable social supports, either family or close friends. A reliable support system ensures that any deviations in the expected course of the withdrawal process will be observed and reported. Because of the nature of alcoholism, family members and other close relations (girlfriends, roommates) often suffer greatly during the course of the active illness. Family members, frustrated and angry by the prior behavior of the patient, may be reluctant to take responsibility for the patient during the withdrawal period, or the home may not be a safe place for detoxification because of the presence of other active drinkers. The physician should first contact a key family member and explore the notion of home detoxification. He will have to decide whether the family needs help before involving them in managing the patient at home. If help is needed, the family should be advised to go to Al-Anon, seek a family counselor, or have the patient detoxified in an inpatient setting.

Mrs G's involvement in Al-Anon enabled her to help Mr G come for help. It also assured the physician that she had a positive support network during the difficult period of Mr G's recovery.

Physician–Patient Relationship

The physician and patient should have a preexisting relationship as the basis for negotiating the methods and conditions of outpatient detoxification. The doctor–patient relationship serves as a cornerstone for the recovery process because, when established, it creates a safe environment in which the patient can learn about sobriety.[3] The physician must be astute, relaxed, knowledgeable, and nonjudgmental about difficulties encountered by the alcoholic patient. In addition, he should educate and offer advice about treatment options: AA, local detoxification centers, employee-assistance programs, and alcohol counselors. Many clinicians face the dilemma of having a doctor–patient relationship inadequate for pursuing ambulatory detoxification safely. This situation occurs most often with new patients in mild withdrawal, but it is also seen with patients who complain that they have "hit bottom," requiring medical attention for their advanced disease.

Mr G's long-term relationship with his clinician provided the trust and setting necessary for him to abstain for one month. His follow-up visits revealed slow resolution of his symptoms and laboratory abnormalities. During daily visits after detoxification, Mr G's physician encouraged him to attend an AA meeting. Mr G replied, "That is for real down and out alcoholics, not me."

The beginning of postdetoxification management starts during the detoxification process. The doctor–patient relationship plays a vital role in negotiating the use of adjunctive support groups to maintain sobriety. Several strategies might help obtain Mr G's agreement to attend a trial meeting of AA at this juncture. These are discussed more fully in Chapter 7.

Pharmacotherapy

Any patient who experiences untoward side effects from alcohol withdrawal should be offered drug therapy. Although a nonpharmacologic approach has been effective in detoxification in inpatient settings,[4] the relatively uncontrolled home environment warrants the use of a sedative in outpatient detoxification. Drug therapy for minor alcohol withdrawal syndromes on an ambulatory basis is relatively simple. Although many sedatives provide relief, benzodiazepines (particularly chlorodiazepoxide and oxazepam) are widely used because of their effectiveness and safety. Chlordiazepoxide has a longer half-life and, therefore, gives a smoother detoxification. Oxazepam is more appropriate when there is severe liver disease because it does not have active metabolites, and elimination of the drug is independent of liver function.[1,2] Other classes of drugs, such as the beta-andrenergic blockers, which may have some use as adjunctive agents in the treatment of alcohol withdrawal, have not been evaluated for outpatient use.[5]

In outpatient detoxification, the health care team must monitor the patient's course closely. Following vital signs is more important in determining the need for tranquilizers than are the patient's subjective feelings. Chlordiazepoxide is given in the office in dosages of 50 mg to 100 mg. Because all benzodiazepines are poorly absorbed intramuscularly, oral therapy is used on an outpatient basis. The patient is observed for an hour or two in the office and then sent home with a companion, with not more than 200 mg chlordiazepoxide, taking 25 mg every four to six hours as needed. The physician assesses the total dose used in the first 24 hours, reevaluates the patient, and if everything is stable, instructs the patient to take half the total initial daily dose on day two (usually 100 mg to 150 mg). The same screening process continues, with daily decreases of 50% in the total dose, that is, 50 mg the third day, and then none. One may substitute diazepam or oxazepam. Chlordiazepoxide 100 mg is equivalent to 20 mg diazepam and 90 mg oxazepam.[6]

Mr. G fared well during an uneventful detoxification taking oxazepam at home. He was seen daily during that time, and on the third visit, time was spent finding an AA meeting for him to try. After much resistance, he agreed to go that night, but to another town where he would not be recognized. Although Mr G saw no reason for frequent visits once his physical symptoms had abated, his physician requested that Mr. G return every one to three weeks during early recovery.

Once the patient is detoxified for the acute symptoms, the process of recovery begins. Many experience prolonged withdrawal symptoms, including insomnia, nervousness, and fearfulness. Tranquilizers should not be used in the treatment of prolonged symptoms, which usually abate over six months. Support, including AA, employee-assistance programs, and alcoholism counseling can circumvent the need for medication during this time.

References

1. Sellers E, Kalant H: Alcohol intoxication and withdrawal. *N Engl J Med* 1976;294: 757–762.
2. Jacobs MS, Sellers E: Emergency management of alcohol withdrawal. *Drug Therapy* (Hospital Edition) April, 1977;28–34.
3. Bean M: Clinical implications of models for recovery from alcoholism. *Adv Alcohol Substance Abuse* 1983;3:91–104.
4. Whitfield C, Thompson G, et al: Detoxification of 1,024 alcoholic patients without psychoactive drugs. *JAMA* 1978;239:1409–1410.
5. Kraus MG, Gottlieb LD, Morwitz RI, Anscher M: Randomized clinical trial of atenolol in patients with alcohol withdrawal. *N Engl J Med* 1985;313:905–909.
6. Clark WD: Alcohol abuse, in Kravis TC, Warner CG (eds): *Emergency Medicine: A Comprehensive Review.* Rockville, Md, Aspen Systems, 1983, pp 517–531.

10
Management of the Alcoholic Inpatient

BOOKER BUSH

The prevalence of alcohol abuse in hospitalized medical patients may range as high as 20% to 40%.[1] The majority of these patients enter the hospital for illnesses not directly related to alcohol abuse, but subsequent withdrawal from alcohol or other alcohol-related problems can complicate the hospital course. If the primary care physician has treated the alcohol abuser as an outpatient, he can use the opportunity of hospitalization to initiate or consolidate long-term treatment of alcohol abuse. Although management of acute withdrawal is the initial issue, the primary care physician must recall that alcoholism is a chronic disease. Just as diabetic ketoacidosis is an acute issue treated over the course of days, the patient must still learn to care for his diabetes for years. Similarly, the physician must be ready to educate and support the alcoholic patient in the long-term management of his disease.

The care offered to patients admitted to a hospital for acute alcoholism can be divided into two parts: detoxification and rehabilitation. Detoxification occurs over a three to ten day period. The pharmacologic therapy includes the use of medications to decrease the symptoms of alcohol withdrawal and to allow the beginning of alcohol education. The ideal program includes frequent meetings for the patient with counselors, physicians, and alcoholics in recovery. Attendance at AA meetings during hospitalization can be a critical part of the treatment. It is especially important that the physician point out to the patient any physical signs and symptoms that are secondary to alcohol abuse. Together they should discuss whether symptoms are permanent or reversible and what the effect of future alcohol intake will be. They should agree on a plan for medical follow-up and an outpatient treatment program, including AA meetings and/or individual counseling. The majority of patients may return home after detoxification and continue as an outpatient, but patients who have a history of relapse or suicidal tendencies or lack the proper home environment may require long-term or rehabilitation hospitalization.

The physician should avoid hospitalizing an alcoholic patient for detoxification in a facility without any alcoholism treatment services because education about alcoholism is an integral part of any treatment for the disease. The patient might prefer to be hospitalized on the medical service of a general hospital for observation and have the symptoms of alcohol withdrawal treated without addressing the alcoholism. Acute medical treatment for alcoholism without confronting the alcoholism and initiating rehabilitative therapy may in fact prolong the course of the disease because it enables the patient to deny the underlying cause of his acute symptoms.

Recognition and Management of Alcohol Withdrawal

A young, single woman is 24 hours postoperative after open reduction of a tibial fracture suffered in an automobile accident. She was the driver. Blood alcohol on admission was 250 mg/dL, although the patient had not appeared inebriated. On examination, she is alert, anxious, but cooperative. She admits to an occasional six-pack of beer. She denies the use of any benzodiazepines or recreational drugs. On physical examination she has a blood pressure of 140/90, pulse of 104, and a temperature of 99°F. The liver is enlarged and tender. Her blood tests are significant for an MCV of 104, an AST of 250, and a GGT of 800. The orthopedist asks you to comment on her abnormal liver function tests and recommend management. The young woman's parents want to speak to you about their concern over her drinking.

Although the elevated transaminases suggest alcoholic hepatitis, the more immediate concern is whether she needs therapy for her alcohol withdrawal. The clinician must differentiate between minor and major withdrawal (discussed in Chapter 4). Minor withdrawal has an excellent prognosis with a variety of therapies. A supportive environment may be adequate for minor withdrawal, but delirium tremens requires parenteral therapy and intensive monitoring. The goal is to detoxify a patient safely and facilitate acceptance of treatment. It is critical that the physician inform the patient that she is being treated for substance addiction.

Treatment of the alcohol withdrawal syndrome is based on many traditions and clinical impressions. In 1838, Romano found that nutrition, liquids, and avoidance of restraints compared favorably to the use of quinine, opium, or bleeding in the treatment of withdrawal.[2] Goldsmith in 1930 found that spinal drainage to decompress brain swelling did not improve survival in alcohol withdrawal.[3] Finally, Gunne in 1957 found that survival was directly proportional to the modesty of therapy given.[4]

The pharmacologic therapy for alcohol withdrawal is based on the use of drugs that show cross-dependence with alcohol. If given in adequate quantities, barbiturates, benzodiazepines, chloral hydrate, and paraldehyde are all effective in suppressing the withdrawal syndrome. Although there are no studies to support the concept, there is general agreement among pharmacologists and clinicians that these agents will also prevent the development of withdrawal symptoms.

Although the phenothiazines have little cross-dependence with alcohol, clinicians continue to find chlorpromazine and haloperidol useful in treating alcohol withdrawal, especially in the therapy of alcoholic hallucinosis. These drugs appear to shorten the period of hospitalization, although several studies have shown that promazine and chlorpromazine do not prevent the development of delirium tremens and that the mortality rate is significantly higher than in patients treated with paraldehyde or chlordiazepoxide.[5]

Treatment for Minor Withdrawal

The benzodiazepines are usually the drugs of first choice in the treatment of minor withdrawal. Chlordiazepoxide is the drug that has been the standard of care for more than 10 years. Its long half-life of 24 to 48 hours is both its strong point and major weakness. The half-life of the drug is even more prolonged with liver disease or in patients over the age of 60. The long duration of action allows for dosing every six hours, but patients are frequently sedated late in the detoxification process, which interferes with education and counseling. Many clinicians favor a benzodiazepine with a shorter half-life, such as oxazepam. Although oxazepam may need to be administered as often as every three to four hours, the lack of sedation late in detoxification and freedom from hepatic excretion make this a good drug for the elderly and other patients with compromised liver function.

At the start of detoxification, the patient should receive a sedating dose of benzodiazepine in amounts equivalent to 100 mg of chlordiazepoxide or 60 mg of oxazepam. This dose may be repeated in one to two hours if sedation is not obtained. Then, 50 mg of chlordiazepoxide every six hours or 30 mg of oxazepam every four hours should be given. For most patients, the dosage should be reduced by one-half every 24 hours. The dosing interval should remain constant while the dose is tapered.

The majority of patients suffering minor withdrawal only require four to five days of pharmacologic therapy. Sleep disturbance and tremulousness may persist, but tachycardia, nausea, and gross tremor should disappear. Persistent withdrawal symptoms should raise the suspicion of chronic benzodiazepine or barbiturate abuse in addition to alcoholism. Because of body size or extent of tolerance, some patients require higher or more frequent dosages of benzodiazepines. Tachycardia and elevated blood pressures are useful, objective signs to determine the need for more or less medication.

Treatment of Major Withdrawal

The treatment of patients with delirium tremens requires aggressive attention to the withdrawal state and careful assessment of associated medical problems. The presence of pneumonia, pancreatitis, or hepatitis places these patients at high risk. They are frequently dehydrated, have vitamin deficiencies, hypokalemia, hypomagnesemia, hypophosphatemia, thrombocytopenia, and acidemia. Such patients should be monitored closely because fluid and respiratory status can change rapidly. Many clinicians consider delirium tremens an indication for monitoring in an intensive care unit. The reduction in mortality over the last decade from 15% to 2% reflects more careful attention to the medical complications of delirium tremens.[6]

The best therapy for delirium tremens is intravenous diazepam. The majority of patients are too ill or confused to tolerate oral medications, and the intramuscular absorption of medications, such as chlordiazepoxide and paraldehyde, is unpredictable. After the patient is placed in a carefully monitored room with respiratory support equipment easily available and good venous access obtained, therapy is begun with 5 to 10 mg of diazepam. This dose is repeated every five minutes until the patient is quiet and sedated. Initial doses of 30 to 80 mg of diazepam are not unusual in these patients. Careful observation should continue, however, since the peak effect of diazepam may occur one to two hours after the initial dose.

If parenteral therapy is not available, the second therapy of choice is paraldehyde, which may be given either orally or by rectal enema. The initial dose of 10 to 20 mL may be repeated every one to two hours until sedation is reached. The major drawback of this therapy (other than its noxious odor) is respiratory depression, which may occur hours after a dose. A comparison of diazepam and paraldehyde for treatment of delirium tremens noted equal efficacy but increased side effects with paraldehyde.[7]

Many clinicians continue to use haloperidol or phenothiazines for the treatment of delirium tremens. Although these medications lower the seizure threshold, withdrawal seizures usually occur before the onset of delirium tremens, and once delirium tremens appears, seizures should no longer be a problem in the majority of patients. Haloperidol and phenothiazines have an advantage over the sedative-hypnotic drugs in that they do not cause respiratory depression. Chlorpromazine in doses of 25 to 100 mg intramuscularly is given to patients under the age of 60. Because of possible hypotension in older patients, haloperidol in doses of 3 to 5 mg intramuscularly is given to those over the age of 60. The dose is repeated every four to six hours on an as-needed basis to keep the patient calm.

Alcohol Withdrawal Seizures

Seizures may occur in the first 48 hours of alcohol withdrawal from either discontinuing or reducing alcohol intake. They are usually generalized and self-limited, but focal seizures may occur as part of alcohol withdrawal. New focal seizures should prompt a search for some other cause, such as subdural hematoma or CNS infections. When the only etiology for a seizure is alcohol, long-term drug therapy with anticonvulsants is not necessary. Cessation of alcohol is essential.

There are few data to support prophylaxis for alcohol withdrawal seizures in patients who have no history of previous seizures, but for those patients with a known seizure disorder or a previous history of withdrawal seizures, oral diphenylhydantoin is effective for prophylaxis.[8] A loading dose is not necessary; 300 mg of diphenylhydantoin given daily is adequate. However, conflicting evidence suggests that, if patients are adequately sedated with benzodiazepines, anticonvulsants may add little protection against seizures.[9] If the patient has only withdrawal seizures, therapy can be discontinued when detoxification is complete.

Nutritional Problems

Although the majority of alcoholics do not have nutritional problems, many who develop alcoholic hepatitis or alcoholic ketoacidosis have specific vitamin and mineral deficiencies, the most common being thiamine deficiency. In its severe form, thiamine deficiency results in Wernicke's encephalopathy with ataxia, ocular palsies, nystagmus, and mental confusion. To avert encephalopathy, the patient should receive 100 mg of intravenous thiamine before any glucose is administered. In lower-risk hospitalized patients, the preferred route of administration is 100 mg of thiamine by mouth or intramuscularly because of the small risk of anaphylaxis with intravenous administration.

Alcohol is a potent magnesium diuretic. Hypomagnesemia will cause hypocalcemia, since magnesium is required both for parathyroid hormone release and its action on bone. A low magnesium level may also exacerbate the effects of thiamine deficiency.[10] If hypomagnesemia is severe, correction can be accomplished over six to 12 hours by replenishing magnesium with 8 to 10 g of magnesium sulfate in a liter of intravenous fluid. If there is no acute metabolic disturbance and the patient is able to eat, there is no need for parenteral supplementation. Those patients unable to eat should receive the daily requirement for magnesium of 200 mg. Two ampules of magnesium sulfate (50%) can be given intramuscularly or intravenously every day.

A special problem in alcoholic patients who are admitted with alcoholic ketoacidosis or severe dehydration is phosphate depletion. Hypophosphatemia is usually due to poor nutrition. As in diabetic ketoacidosis, hypophosphatemia will become evident after intravenous glucose administration increases the cellular uptake of phosphate. The nadir occurs 48 to 72 hours into therapy for the ketoacidosis. When phosphate levels drop below 1 mg/dL, rhabdomyolysis and hemolytic anemia can occur. The safest method of repletion is to give oral phosphate. If the oral route is not available, intravenous potassium phosphate is administered.

Patients who are phosphate depleted will need 0.1 mmol/kg body weight. Potassium phosphate contain 3 mmol of phosphate/ml. In a 70 kg patient, 2 mL of K-phos given intravenously over six hours is adequate. Serum levels of phosphate must be monitored regularly, since serum levels do not reflect intracellular stores and equilibrium is reached in 12 to 24 hours.

Investigational Therapies

There are a number of randomized, controlled trials describing the use of betablockers or clonidine in association with benzodiazepines for the treatment of alcohol withdrawal.[11,12] These drugs are effective in suppressing the autonomic discharge that accompanies alcohol withdrawal and, in a small number of patients, have compared favorably with the use of sedative hypnotics alone. One drawback is that progression to delirium tremens has been quite frequent in the beta-blocker treatment groups.[13]

General Care of the Patient

As the consultant called to see the 25-year-old woman recuperating from open reduction of a tibial fracture, the physician knows the patient has tolerance to alcohol because she appeared sober despite a level of 250 mg/dL of ethanol. In addition, she is anxious, tachycardic, hypertensive, and has an enlarged and tender liver. To initiate therapy, the physician investigates her previous history of alcohol withdrawal and her use of benzodiazepines or other sedatives. The physician performs a thorough neurologic examination and attempts to evaluate her nutritional status.

If evaluation reveals that this is her first experience with alcohol withdrawal, the physician should inform her of her tolerance to alcohol, the mild withdrawal she is experiencing, and her abnormal liver tests. A reasonable treatment plan would include benzodiazepines for her withdrawal and an alcohol-education program of visits to hospital AA meetings if available, visits by AA members, and one-on-one counseling. The physician should monitor her magnesium, phosphate, and liver transaminase levels during hospitalization. The consultant should recommend an aftercare program with AA or some other alcohol program on an outpatient basis. The parents should be referred to Al-Anon. Family therapy might also be helpful.

The patient may choose to reject much of the plan. However, it is important to present the diagnosis and prognosis both to the patient and to the family. The consultant should be specific that the pharmacologic therapy is for her minor withdrawal, so that her alcohol abuse is a primary issue. Frequently, such a hospitalization proves to be a first, important step toward recovery.

References

1. Ramnik B, Stewart MA, Guze SB: Prevalence of alcoholism among general ward patients. *Am J Psychiatry* 1968;125:133–136.
2. Ware J: Early contributions to the study of delirium tremens. *Ann Med Hist* 1941;3:128–139.
3. Goldsmith H: Spinal drainage in alcoholic deliria and other acute alcoholic psychoses. *Am J Psychiatry* 1930;87:255–265.
4. Gunne L: Treatment of delirium tremens. *Nord Med* 1957;57:703–706.
5. Gross MM, Lewis E, Hastey J: Acute alcohol withdrawal syndrome, in Kissin B, Begleiter H (eds): *Biology of Alcoholism*. New York: Plenum Press, 1974, vol 3.

6. Naranjo CA, Sellers EM: Clinical assessment and pharmacotherapy of the alcohol withdrawal syndrome, in Galanter, M (ed): *Recent Developments in Alcoholism*. New York, Plenum Press, 1986, vol 4.
7. Thompson WL, Johnson AD, Maddrey WL: Diazepam and paraldehyde in the treatment of severe delirium tremens. Ann Intern Med 1975;82:175–180.
8. Sampliner R, Iber FL: Diphenylhydantoin control of alcohol withdrawal seizures. *JAMA* 1974;230:1430–1432.
9. Rothstein E: Prevention of alcohol withdrawal seizures: The roles of diphenylhydantoin and chlordiazepoxide. *Am J Psychiatry* 1973;130:1381–1382.
10. Zieve L: Influence of magnesium deficiency on the utilization of thiamine. *Ann NY Acad Sci* 1969;162:732–743.
11. Bjorkquist SE: Clonidine in alcohol withdrawal. *Acta Psychiatr Scand* 1975;52: 256–260.
12. Kraus ML, et al: Randomized clinical trial of atenolol in patients with alcohol withdrawal. *N Engl J Med* 1985;313:905–909.
13. Jacob MS: Propranolol-associated confused states during alcohol withdrawal. *J Clin Psychopharmacol* 1983;3:185–191.

Part IV
Resources in the Community and Workplace

This section describes two community resources with which the primary care physician should be familiar: Alcoholics Anonymous and employee-assistance programs. Many patients will achieve sobriety by working with their primary physician in conjunction with AA or employee-assistance programs without recourse to any other specialized program.

In the chapter on AA, Stephen O'Neill and Henrietta Barnes describe the history and organization of AA, with particular attention to what a patient should expect when first attending a meeting. The self-help nature of the groups and the AA program for personal growth are explained in clinical terms. After outlining specific steps for referring a patient to AA, the authors discuss some precepts of AA that may be useful in office practice.

Although employee-assistance programs are not as universally available as AA, Diana Chapman Walsh points out that about 12% of the work force has access to some form of employee-assistance program. Dr. Walsh acknowledges that a variety of programs falls under the rubric of employee-assistance programs and urges the practitioner to be aware of the strengths and limitations of any program in which a patient is involved. Some of the concepts of employee-assistance programs may be applicable to office practice, and the coordinated efforts of the staff of employee-assistance programs and primary care physicians can result in more appropriate, comprehensive care for the alcoholic worker/patient.

Some patients need more intensive forms of treatment for alcoholism. Primary care physicians may have difficulty staying informed about the various alcoholism treatment programs available in their communities. For this reason it is often helpful to identify one person in the field of alcoholism, such as a social worker or counselor, who can act as a resource for referrals. This person not only will have current knowledge of various treatment programs but also can act as a personal contact for the patient during the referral process.

Treatment programs for alcoholism can be divided into inpatient and outpatient resources. Inpatient programs include detoxification and rehabilitation. Detoxification centers are either free-standing or hospital-affiliated. Their short-term programs, usually less than a week, provide for a safe detoxification with or without medication. Although they do offer some minimal education about alcoholism and some assistance with aftercare planning, their main focus is the acute withdrawal period. In contrast, rehabilitation programs are designed to help alcoholics establish sobriety, learn about their alcoholism, and initiate changes in behavior. Most rehabilitation programs use individual counseling, group, and family therapy. The length of rehabilitation programs, usually two to four weeks, reflects the reimbursement schedules of health insurance policies as much as the natural history of recovery. The degree of aftercare planning is an important consideration, especially for patients who may attend a rehabilitation program outside their own communities.

For patients who require prolonged supervision, there are halfway houses. Some of these residential programs emphasize finding a job and maintaining contact with the rest of society. Others are built on the model of a therapeutic community in which the long-term group interactions play a role in the recovery process.

Outpatient alcoholism programs offer a wide variety of services. The type of service usually reflects the philosophy of the particular program: those that are psychotherapeutically oriented offer intense individual or group therapy; community outreach programs operate walk-in services, drop-in centers, or educational sessions. The staffing patterns (health professionals or recovered people) and the sources of funding (fee-for-service versus government grants) often dictate the approach of any particular program. Some outpatient treatment centers serve particular subpopulations: women, adolescents, multiple drug users, or homosexuals. In addition, many communities have specialized programs, such as those for people convicted of driving while intoxicated.

In evaluating a program, the primary care physician must keep in mind that no one program has proven more effective than another. However, when referring an alcoholic patient to a general social service or mental health unit, it is important to ensure that some staff members have expertise in dealing with the treatment of alcoholism. Until further data are available on the efficacy of one form of treatment versus another, the decision about where to refer a patient remains a combination of clinical judgment (evaluation of patient's prior treatment and current needs), external logistics (type of insurance, need for child care), and availability.

11
Alcoholics Anonymous

STEPHEN F. O'NEILL and HENRIETTA N. BARNES

AA is too religious; I don't believe in all the God business.

The meetings are depressing; the speakers talk about all their problems from drinking. I'm not that badly off.

AA is only for real down-and-out alcoholics. I'm not even sure I have a problem.

I'm not the type to join a group; I could never talk in front of all those people.

These reactions, familiar to any physician who has tried to discuss Alcoholics Anonymous (AA) with a patient, often preclude any meaningful referral to AA meetings. Do they represent accurate perceptions of AA, or are they simply manifestations of patients' denial? The answer is probably a combination of both. AA is as effective as more formal treatment modalities but may not be the best therapy for all alcoholics.[1] Understanding AA can help the physician determine which patients are most likely to benefit and how to make an effective referral. When medical therapy is undertaken, patients expect their physicians to describe what the therapy will entail, its risks, the degree of discomfort, and the potential benefits. Although medical education has given most physicians familiarity with common diagnostic and therapeutic procedures, physicians do not have a similar grasp of the therapy in question here: Alcoholics Anonymous.

The Organization of Alcoholics Anonymous

AA is an international federation of self-help groups dedicated to the sole purpose of helping the alcoholic who wishes to stop drinking and achieve sobriety.[2] Founded in 1935 by an alcoholic stockbroker and an alcoholic physician (the legendary Bill W and Dr Bob of AA lore), the organization has grown to an estimated one million active members and some 48,000 groups worldwide.[3]

Bill W and Dr Bob achieved sobriety through mutual support. They then directed their energies toward helping alcoholics on the wards of Cleveland,

Ohio, hospitals to stop drinking. Their experiences were formalized as the Twelve Steps of AA, which provide guidelines for the personal growth necessary to achieve a stable recovery. As the organization grew, it developed, for its own preservation, a parallel set of guidelines, The Twelve Traditions. These tenets assured that AA would not affiliate with other organizations, espouse no cause other than helping an individual achieve sobriety, and never accept outside funding or charge fees. The insistence on anonymity at all levels prevented group leaders from using their positions for personal gain. With the exception of some paid secretarial help, AA is staffed entirely by recovered alcoholic members of AA who volunteer their time. Whereas this independent, nonprofessional stance has enabled AA to appeal to a very diverse population, it has made some physicians reluctant to recommend AA to their patients.[4]

Each autonomous AA group sponsors a weekly meeting. The character of the group usually reflects (1) the ethnic and socioeconomic status of the surrounding community or (2) a special, common interest, such as sexual preference, profession, or addiction to other drugs. There are three types of meetings: open, closed, and beginners' meetings.

Open meetings, available to anyone interested in alcoholism, are directed at people new to the AA program or those returning after a relapse. The format usually consists of several speakers, recovered members from a different AA group who tell their "drunkalogue" (an often wry and humorous account of their troubles with drinking and their recovery through the AA program). Occasionally, open meetings are structured as discussions, moderated by the chairperson of the group. In each meeting, there is a coffee break for socializing, handing out AA literature, or celebrating a member's anniversary of one or more years of sobriety.

Closed meetings may be attended by any member of AA, in theory any person who desires to stop drinking. In actuality, closed meetings generally have a stable core membership and function as leaderless support groups. Because closed meetings attract members more secure in their sobriety, discussions often revolve around issues of personal growth in recovery rather than on techniques for not drinking.

At beginners' meetings, veteran AA members outline the AA program for newcomers. By describing their own experiences in first coming to AA, the veteran members anticipate the fears, anxieties, and sense of isolation that may paralyze the newcomer. Offers to provide phone numbers or to accompany the newcomer to another AA meeting promote an aura of acceptance. Beginners' meetings usually precede an open meeting.

In addition to the public AA meetings, there is an informal network of relationships among recovered AA members. This network provides emotional support, a nondrinking social milieu, and more concrete services (such as helping an actively drinking member obtain medical help). AA also sponsors regional and national conferences and retreats.

The Theoretical Basis of Alcoholics Anonymous

The subtle complexities of the AA program defy any simple description.[5] However, the wealth of anecdotes and personal testament that form the mystique of AA should not obscure the fact that AA has developed a logical program for personal growth and group involvement.

The two basic tenets of AA are that alcoholism is a disease and that abstinence is necessary for recovery. Although the AA assertion that alcoholism is an "allergy to alcohol" does not correspond to the strict medical definition of an allergic reaction, in the broader sense, the concept of alcoholism as a disease is similar to many physicians' understanding of chronic disease: a progressive, often fatal, condition with exacerbations and remissions that can be arrested but not cured. While clearly stating that alcoholism is not caused by moral failure or lack of will power, AA recognizes that alcoholism creates spiritual and emotional, as well as physical, problems and that recovery must address all three areas. Although some early-stage alcoholics do resume drinking without apparent problems,[6,7] AA's insistence on abstinence reflects both the experiences of AA members who have had serious problems with alcohol[6] and the inability to predict which alcoholics might be able to resume drinking safely in the future.

The Group Process

AA meetings function as leaderless self-help groups. Since it is a program of attraction, not coercion,[8] AA must offer something positive and appealing to prospective members. What it offers is a fellowship of sober alcoholics, whose concern with not drinking parallels the alcoholic's previous preoccupation with drinking, and the hope of recovery through participation in the program.

The format of an AA group allows for increasing degrees of involvement. The newly sober alcoholic needs an accepting environment, supportive of his efforts to stay sober, without complex personal interaction. The newcomer may sit in the back of the meeting without any obligation to speak or participate. Cognizant of the newcomer's shame, vulnerability, and ambivalence, the veteran AA member may greet him, share his own first reactions to AA, perhaps offer his phone number, and not ask anything about the newcomer. Initially, the suggestions for the newly sober alcoholic are simple and direct and are often couched in catchy slogans designed to penetrate his postdetoxification dementia: "Don't drink; go to meetings." "Ninety meetings in 90 days." "Easy does it." "One day at a time."[2] The underlying assumption is that the way to maintain sobriety in this early, tenuous period is to immerse oneself in a supportive network of sober alcoholics and avoid stresses that could lead to drinking. "Don't get hungry, angry, lonely, tired (HALT)"—all states that mimic withdrawal and can lead to relapse. During this period, the newcomer may identify with the experience of a speaker, an event that many AA members mark as the turning point in their recovery.[9] Daily attendance at meetings also helps separate the alcoholic from a social system that may have condoned his drinking and from a family that needs time to adjust to the alcoholic's sobriety.

After a few months of sobriety, the alcoholic is encouraged to become more involved in the program. Although many people never participate formally in AA, those who do tend to have better outcomes than those who attend irregularly.[1,6,7] Whether this reflects the success of the program or self-selection of a healthier population is unclear, but a patient's involvement in AA can provide useful prognostic information for his monitoring physician. Increased commitment usually takes the form of affiliating with one particular group and finding a sponsor. The sponsor, a veteran member with at least a year of sobriety, offers guidance and support, including confrontation if the newcomer's behavior indicates he may drink again. The sponsor's most powerful influence may be as a role model of an alcoholic who has achieved a successful sobriety. For the sponsor, the interaction provides a reminder of his own pain in early sobriety and reaffirms the value of his own recovery.[10] The inherent problem in the sponsor-"pigeon" partnership is that often the alcoholic's loneliness and need place overwhelming demands on an individual relationship. For this reason, AA emphasizes the necessity of belonging to a group, which can provide more constant support than any single individual.[11,12]

As his sobriety progresses, the new member may join more veteran members on speaking engagements to other groups. This pivotal experience allows someone whose own sobriety is still tenuous to reach out and inspire others with his "drunkalogue." In return, he receives the audience's acceptance and appreciation of his public declaration, "My name is Joe, and I am an alcoholic." The reciprocal nature of this interaction epitomizes AA philosophy that the newest AA member, suffering, confused, and vulnerable, has something positive to give the group and that, conversely, the most veteran member still needs to be reminded of his continued vulnerability to alcohol.[12]

The Twelve Steps

The Twelve Steps embody AA's principles for recovery from alcoholism. To the medical profession, they are most understandable as a quasireligious expression of the process of change seen in psychotherapy.[10] The fact that the word "alcohol(ic)" appears only in the first and twelfth steps underscores AA's contention that the main work of recovery is not abstinence but a restructuring of the alcoholic's personality.

The explicitly religious language of the Twelve Steps engenders both inspiration in AA members and criticism from skeptical outsiders. AA has attempted to defuse the religious language by posing the Twelve Steps as suggestions and qualifying references to God with the phrase "as we understood Him."[5] Many AA members use their AA group as their source of authority or "Higher Power." Others maintain a more traditionally dogmatic belief system. Understanding the psychologic basis of the Twelve Steps and appreciating the enormous variability of religious tone among AA groups can enable a physician to assess whether a

TABLE 11.1. Twelve suggested steps of Alcoholics Anonymous.

1. We admitted we were powerless over alcohol—that our lives had become unmanageable.
2. Came to believe that a Power greater than ourselves could restore us to sanity.
3. Made a decision to turn our will and our lives over to the care of God as we understood Him.
4. Made a searching and fearless moral inventory of ourselves.
5. Admitted to God, to ourselves and to another human being the exact nature of our wrongs.
6. Were entirely ready to have God remove all these defects of character.
7. Humbly asked Him to remove our shortcomings.
8. Made a list of all persons we had harmed, and became willing to make amends to them all.
9. Made direct amends to such people wherever possible, except when to do so would injure them or others.
10. Continued to take personal inventory and when we were wrong promptly admitted it.
11. Sought through prayer and meditation to improve our conscious contact with God as we understood Him, praying only for knowledge of His will for us and the power to carry that out.
12. Having had a spiritual awakening as the result of these steps, we tried to carry this message to alcoholics, and to practice these principles in all our affairs.

patient's objections to the religious nature of AA reflect incompatibility with a particular group or represent an aspect of denial.

In broad outline, the Twelve Steps (Table 11.1) involve accepting the diagnosis and its implications, believing that recovery is possible, undergoing a period of self-exploration, and finally translating this self-knowledge into appropriate interpersonal behavior. The first three steps parallel the beginning of a psychotherapeutic relationship, in which the problem is articulated and defined, help is requested, and a relationship with an authority figure is established. Steps four through eleven encompass the main work of recovery. They address the paralyzing guilt and remorse that many alcoholics experience in early recovery and provide a way for the alcoholic to take increasing responsibility for his life. These steps parallel the religious process of confession, absolution, and penance. AA members use the steps in different ways: some adhere to them literally, whereas others use them more loosely as guidelines for sober living.[10]

The twelfth step is the keystone of the program, for it reinforces the work of the previous steps by giving a positive altruistic meaning to the painful experience of alcoholism. Literally, the twelfth step work involves helping the actively drinking alcoholic in positive ways, such as accompanying him to an AA meeting or helping him get medical care. Implicit in twelfth step work is the message that the sober alcoholic can identify with the drinker's suffering and that there is hope for recovery through the AA program. In doing twelfth step work, the alcoholic not only provides hope to alcoholics who are still drinking but also develops an improved sense of his own self-worth.

Length of participation in AA is variable. For some, affiliation is lifelong as AA becomes their primary social network. Others find the program's insistence that all problems stem from an individual's drinking to be restrictive once their sobriety is firmly established. There is some debate about whether AA is most effective for achieving early recovery or maintaining long-term sobriety.[10,13] Since newly sober alcoholics have very similar needs, that is, abstinence and support, AA's rigid but comprehensive prescriptions for how to stay sober can be very effective for those patients who avail themselves of the program. AA appears less effective in addressing the diverse needs and problems of alcoholics with several years of sobriety.[14]

Referring Patients to Alcoholics Anonymous

Mrs Smith, a 42-year-old bookkeeper with peptic ulcer disease, acknowledges frequent criticisms from her family about her difficulty in controlling her drinking. Because she has recently been put on probation at work for frequent tardiness, she reluctantly agrees to get some help for her "alcohol problem."

Ms Fountain is a 24-year-old graduate student who complains of insomnia and anxiety. She states that she has been drinking more heavily since she broke up with her boyfriend two months ago. Her father and maternal grandfather both had alcoholism.

Most physicians would agree that Mrs Smith has alcoholism and that a referral to AA would be appropriate, but would AA be useful for Ms Fountain? Her family history and drinking pattern put her at high risk for developing alcoholism. A referral to AA may be helpful diagnostically for physician and patient. Ms Fountain, referred to AA to learn about the disease, may discover that some of her symptoms are indicative of alcoholism. A subsequent discussion of her reaction to AA may yield further data about the role of alcohol in her life.

Although AA does not define its program as "treatment,"[2] its diversity and accessibility make it an appropriate form of therapy for most patients with alcoholism. However, there are some types of patients who may have difficulty availing themselves of the program. Patients with poorly developed social skills or difficulty forming relationships may not be able to tolerate the interpersonal interaction in AA. With adequate assurance about the anonymity of AA and the usefulness of just listening to the speakers, some of these patients may benefit from peripheral involvement. Patients who require psychiatric medications face a special problem: they may be criticized for their use of psychotropic drugs. Although AA has no formal policy against medications, some members' negative attitudes about medications may undercut their therapeutic value. Occasionally, patients with very early stage alcoholism may not be able to identify with the experiences of AA members. A discussion of any similarities in drinking patterns, rather than the individual consequences (as well as a referral to a beginner's meeting) may enable such patients to participate.

Few physicians would say to a patient, "You've got an abnormal heart rhythm; go find yourself a cardiologist." Yet the admonition, "You drink too much; why don't you go to AA," is a familiar response to the alcoholic patient. In order to have a patient accept any referral, the physician must convey knowledge of and respect for the person or agency to whom the referral is made, and the patient must not experience the referral as rejection. Successful referral to AA requires that the physician address these same issues.

A specific recommendation to attend an AA meeting requires some knowledge of AA meetings in the patient's community or at least access to that knowledge. Meeting lists are published by the local AA Central Service Office in most metropolitan areas and are available in bulk for a nominal fee. Giving a patient a booklet, discussing which meetings he plans to attend, and even writing a prescription for attendance at AA convey the physician's seriousness about the referral. If the physician has attended an AA meeting, the personal experience enhances the credibility of the referral as well as understanding of the program. Practicing internists and medical residents both rated attendance at an AA meeting as one of the most valuable aspects of a seminar on alcoholism.[15]

Finding an AA member to accompany a patient to his first meeting can allay some of his initial anxiety. Because of their commitment to twelfth step work, many recovered alcoholics are eager to help in this way. A screening alcohol history on all patients, plus a sign in the office waiting room, may help identify sober alcoholics in the physician's own practice. Often the AA Central Service Office can provide a contact in the patient's community. When a physician offers to accompany a patient to a meeting,[5] the doctor's seriousness about the importance of AA will almost always mobilize patients to attend on their own.

The physician needs to match the urgency of referral with the seriousness of the problem. In referring patients whose diagnosis is unclear or who have not yet accepted the diagnosis of alcoholism, the physician may suggest they attend three to four different meetings and then return to discuss their impressions. For other alcoholic patients, the recommendation that they attend at least one meeting a day until the next visit (a paraphrase of AA's "90 meetings in 90 days") is likely to result in attendance at a few meetings at least. The goal is to expose the patient to a sufficient number of meetings to allow him to make an informed judgment about the usefulness of AA for himself.

Discussing a patient's reaction to AA will help ensure continued participation. The patient needs to understand that reactions to AA, be they positive or negative, and continued involvement in the program are matters of concern to the physician. If the physician maintains the posture that the patient need not like or enjoy AA in order to benefit from it, much as a patient might tolerate the side effects of a beneficial medication, the patient may continue in AA despite minor criticisms. If there are more serious incompatibilities with a particular group, the physician should encourage the patient to try other groups. Concrete knowledge of AA can help the physician evaluate whether the patient's reaction represents denial. For instance, the common complaint that AA meetings and the speakers are depressing is easily countered by anyone who has experienced the warmth of a meeting and heard speakers talk about not only their problems with alcohol but their successes with recovery.

Using the Precepts of Alcoholics Anonymous in the Office

The collective enthusiasm of AA members about the possibility of recovery and the personal worth of each alcoholic contrasts sharply with the pessimism and negative attitudes that have prevailed in the medical profession.[16,17] What can physicians learn from AA that will enable them to provide more effective care to alcoholic patients?

First, AA is very clear about the limits of individual responsibility for both the alcoholic and his caregivers. Just as the alcoholic acknowledges that he is "powerless over alcohol," so too his friends in AA recognize that they cannot control his alcoholism or his recovery. Exacerbations are common and unpredictable, and the emotional needs of alcoholics can be overwhelming. The inability to meet all of these needs reflects the protean nature of the disease and not the inadequacies of a caregiver. If the physician does not expect to cure the alcoholic but only to decrease suffering by enabling the patient to help himself, the physician will avoid much of the frustration and disappointment that are inevitable when the patient's demands escalate and relapse ensues.

AA members, through their meetings, provide safety, education, and hope. In the context of the office, the physician can do the same. If there are realistic expectations, patients' relapses will not be perceived as personal failures and each new alcoholic patient will be accepted as a challenge for medical management. Knowledge of AA and understanding its precepts can result in more effective referrals and make working with alcoholics an enjoyable and challenging experience rather than a discouraging and frustrating one.

References

1. Baekeland F: Evaluation of treatment methods in chronic alcoholism, in Kissin B, Begleiter H (eds): *The Biology of Alcoholism*. New York, Plenum Press, 1977, vol 5, *Treatment and Rehabilitation of the Chronic Alcoholic*, pp 385–440.
2. Alcoholics Anonymous World Services, Inc., PO Box 459, Grand Central Station, New York, NY.
3. *Alcoholics Anonymous*, ed 3. New York, Alcoholics Anonymous World Services, 1976.
4. Kalb M, Propper MS: The future of alcohology: Craft or science? *Am J Psychiatry* 1976;133(6):641–645.
5. Bean M, Whitfield C, Williams K: *Alcoholics Anonymous*. Unpublished.
6. Vaillant GE: *The Natural History of Alcoholism: Causes, Patterns, and Paths to Recovery*. Cambridge, Mass, Harvard University Press, 1983.
7. Polich JM, Armor DJ, Braiker HB: *The Course of Alcoholism: Four Years after Treatment*. New York, John Wiley and Sons, 1981.
8. Clark WD: Alcoholism: Blocks to diagnosis and treatment. *Am J Med* 1981;71: 275–286.
9. Cutler DF: Personal communication, 1983.
10. Bean MH: Alcoholics Anonymous. *Psychiatr Ann* 1975;5(2):7–61.

11. Vaillant GH: Dangers of psychotherapy in the treatment of alcoholism, in Bean MH, Zinberg NE (eds): *Dynamic Approaches to the Understanding and Treatment of Alcoholism*. New York, Free Press, 1981, pp 36–54.
12. Alibrandi LA: The folk psychotherapy of Alcoholics Anonymous, in Zimberg S, Wallace J, Blume SB (eds). *Practical Approaches to Alcoholism Therapy*. New York, Plenum Press, 1978.
13. Curlee J: How a therapist can use Alcoholics Anonymous. *Ann NY Acad Sci* 1974; 233:137–143.
14. Bean MH: Denial and the psychological complications of alcoholism, in Bean MH, Zinberg NE (eds): *Dynamic Approaches to the Understanding and Treatment of Alcoholism*. New York, Free Press, 1981, pp 55–96.
15. Warburg MM, Cleary PD, Rohman M, et al: Diagnosis and management of alcoholism: A survey of medical residents. *J Med Educ* 1987;62(6):497–503.
16. Fisher JC, et al: Physicians and alcoholics: Effects of medical training on attitudes toward alcoholics. *J Stud Alcohol* 1975;36:949.
17. Chappel J: Physician attitudes: Effect on treatment of chemically dependent patients. *JAMA* 1977;237:2318.

12
Employee-assistance Programs and the Primary Care Practitioner

DIAN CHAPMAN WALSH

The two-way street connecting work and health has long been recognized—if not fully understood—by occupational physicians whose clinical isolation goes back at least a century. Alcoholism treatment has also drifted in a medical backwater, although some of the early, successful medical efforts to deal with drinking problems were undertaken in the 1930s by occupational physicians at Eastman Kodak and E.I. DuPont de Nemours. The strategy for confronting and treating the alcoholic that was developed at that time has become the cornerstone of what is now known as an employee-assistance program or EAP.[1-4] These programs are expanding rapidly as economic, political, and social forces, which are transforming both occupational medicine and the treatment of alcoholism and alcohol abuse, converge in the workplace.

An employee-assistance program can be defined generically as a set of company and/or union policies and procedures that identify and respond to problems employees are having with (1) alcohol, (2) other substances, or (3) other life stresses that may interfere directly or indirectly with acceptable job performance.[5] In spite of the tremendous variation from one program to another, there is general consensus in the field about the elements and principles that characterize an EAP.[6] These are summarized in Figure 12.1.

Following the pioneering work at Kodak and DuPont, occupational alcoholism programs (the precursors of the modern EAPs) spread at a measured pace through the 1940s, 1950s, and 1960s. In the mid-1970s the numbers of programs under various auspices began to increase, partially due to an explicit federal government policy to foster their growth. Many programs broadened their scope of concern from alcohol and drugs to a whole range of problems experienced by employees and, occasionally, their families. At present, there are said to be thousands of such programs and however skeptical one may be about what these estimates accept as a "program," there can be little doubt that the EAP field has been rapidly expanding.[6] Programs exist in small and large unions and in every type of work setting, including over 50% of Fortune 500 companies, a proportion expected to increase to 70% by 1990.[7] Approximately 12% of workers in the United States are thought to have access to such programs (although "access" covers a broad spectrum of possibilities).

Assumptions

1. Problem identification through supervisor because of impaired job performance.
2. Alcoholism recognized as a treatable medical problem.
3. Disciplinary procedures suspended temporarily while employee enrolled in assistance program.
4. Improved job performance the principal criterion for judging success.

Components

1. Written policy and procedures.
2. Labor and management cooperate in program development and operation.
3. Program personnel refer employees to mental health counselors for diagnostic judgment.
4. Supervisors and shop stewards become oriented to their responsibilities.
5. Program information is conveyed to the work force.
6. Health insurance is extended to cover treatment.
7. Total confidentiality is assured.

Issues

1. Approach

(Narrow) ↓ (Wide)

- –Alcohol program only
- –EAP, and alcohol program, separate but complementary
- –EAP, including alcohol program

2. Function

(Limited) ↓ (Comprehensive)

- –Consultation and outreach
- –Assessment and referral
- –Diagnosis and general referral
- –Diagnostic treatment

3. Location

(Internal) ↓ (External)

- –Inhouse
  - –Medical
  - –Personnel
  - –Other
- –Contract with
  - –Consultant
  - –Consortium
  - –Treatment center(s)

FIGURE 12.1. Employee Assistance Programs: An Overview. Adapted from U.S. Department of Health and Human Services, *Fourth Special Report to the U.S. Congress on Alcohol and Health* (Washington, D.C.: U.S. Government Printing Office, 1981: 125), Reprinted from Walsh, D.C., "Employee Assistance Programs," *Milbank Memorial Fund Quarterly/Health and Society 60* (3, Summer), 1982: 496–497.

Investment by the business sector in these programs reflects awareness of the economic, social, medical—and human—burden associated with alcohol and substance abuse, together with the hope that afflicted employees can be treated successfully and resume productive lives. A number of published studies purport to substantiate this hope, but none withstands critical scrutiny regarding the validity and reliability of its findings.[8] Studies have assessed whether changes in drinking behavior, changes in job performance, cost reductions, or combinations of these results can be attributed to enrollment of employees in job-based alcoholism programs. However, serious methodologic flaws make it impossible to point with certainty to evidence that these programs benefit their clients or sponsors.[9]

In the absence of convincing scientific evidence that the investment is warranted, it would be puzzling to see so many employers supporting EAPs were it not for two mitigating factors: (1) the level of investment is minimal in all but a very few instances (usually businesses where public safety is a concern, eg, transportation), and (2) the programs serve a variety of ancillary purposes. Employees like them, the union wants them, they are viewed as good for recruitment and morale, they enhance the company's image, or they are being developed as a product line. When this is the case, it is not essential that they actually reduce drinking, improve productivity, or save money. Moreover, most business managers have seen firsthand the devastation alcohol can cause and have an intuitive sense that an EAP ought to be good for the company and its employees.

Underlying Philosophy

The logic that has been developed to support an EAP weaves together an administrative and a therapeutic rationale. It starts with the concept of alcoholism as a disease of denial and uses the leverage of job loss to break down the drinker's denial so he can be coaxed into treatment. To complement this therapeutic thinking, the administrative rationale maintains that the employer has no right to intervene in an employee's private life but has an obligation to other employees, customers, and stockholders to document and redress unsatisfactory or declining job performance. The final thread holding this fabric together is the belief that drinking problems will be visible in chronic tardiness, absenteeism, and other decrements in performance. Although seldom recognized, this logic is flawed by a basic contradiction: It views the job as the final lifeline that the problem drinker will refuse to release when the rest of life has disintegrated (hence the presumed power of job leverage) but, simultaneously, construes the workplace as a setting where drinking problems will surface early and clearly in declining or unacceptable job performance. In fact, some of the literature suggests that alcoholic employees are able to hide their drinking and turn in superior job performances for a long time after other aspects of their lives have deteriorated.

Employee-assistance Programs and Primary Care Practice

Why should a primary care physician concerned with problem drinking learn about employee-assistance programs? First, some of the principles and tactics evolved over the years in the workplace may be translatable to clinical settings. The *Fifth Special Report to Congress* from the National Institute on Alcohol Abuse and Alcoholism (NIAAA) noted that industry-based programs seem to be challenging the shibboleth that treatment for alcoholism has to be entirely voluntary in order to succeed.[7] A blending of confrontation, coercion, and support are at the center of the employee-assistance philosophy. Some of these principles are applicable to clinical practice, indeed the growing interest in intervention work in clinical settings builds very directly on the EAP experience.

Second, primary care physicians should know when problem-drinking patients are experiencing pressures at work. The threat of job loss has the potential to be a positive, decisive factor in breaking down denial. Even without overt pressure from a patient's employer, a clinician can use problems on the job as a motivating factor. Physicians should also be alert to potentially negative pressures at work—social pressures to drink to conform with co-workers' behavior or job stresses and worries that encourage some workers to drink. A treatment plan to help patients develop effective strategies must account for these pressures in the environment where they spend most of their time.

As another factor in the evaluation of the situation, clinicians need information on what treatments are covered in the employee benefit package through the EAP. Often this information plays a decisive role in treatment planning. Although there is no convincing scientific evidence favoring care rendered in residential programs,[10] inpatient care is more fully covered in employee benefit plans than are outpatient alternatives. Most large employers provide disability insurance to replace wages during a long hospital stay, an additional incentive to select inpatient care.

Finally, in the realm of evaluation, alcoholic patients may be clients of an established employee-assistance program whose efforts ought to complement (or at least not contradict) those of the primary care practitioner. Personnel staffing such programs vary widely in their professional backgrounds and sophistication. Psychiatrists and occupational physicians may be involved if the drinking employee is a high-level manager. For the remainder of the workforce, medical input is less common. EAPs are staffed by clinical psychologists, social workers, health educators, recovered alcoholics, and lay managers. Programs differ greatly in diagnoses, and workforces vary. The implication for outside clinicians is that they should be wary of diagnostic labels their patients may have picked up on passing through at least some EAPs. The crisis situation in which some clients find their way into the EAP is often not conducive to a thoughtful diagnostic workup.

At the other end of the treatment continuum, from the primary physician's perspective, EAPs provide a mechanism to provide aftercare or follow-up for a patient who needs ongoing monitoring or support at work. In some companies, there is a highly structured probationary period where EAP clients are insulated from the disciplinary process as long as they continue to cooperate. Cooperation may be attending a prescribed number of AA meetings each week and reporting back, or it may be a less formal arrangement where the EAP administrator or counselor is available as a sounding board or sympathetic listener.

Another consideration for the period following a course of treatment is whether a patient's employer can arrange job accommodations to ease reentry into the workplace or remove some of the pressures that may have been part of the original problem. High-risk jobs for recovered alcoholics are those involving travel, handling alcohol, or involvement in a heavy drinking subculture. The night shift in a manufacturing organization can provide a haven for an actively drinking employee but create a hell for one struggling to sustain a fragile recovery. Although moving employees around is not a simple matter, the federal Rehabilitation Act stipulates that employers must make "reasonable accommodations" for employees who declare a handicap (and alcoholism is defined specifically as a handicap encompassed by the law). For patients convinced that their jobs will deter recovery, this is an avenue that clinicians might help them explore.

Finally, for clinicians with an interest in research it is worth mentioning that because EAPs are gaining acceptance rapidly and because they create pressures and incentives unique to the workplace, some studies should be carried out in these natural settings. Maintaining contact with research subjects over a period of months or years is made easier when the study is being conducted in concert with a company or a union.

Despite the constructive ways a physician might interact with a patient's employer, it is crucial to underscore the issue of confidentiality. Leaders in the EAP field have been striving to articulate a clear and fair policy governing how to handle sensitive information.[11] However, the threats to confidentiality are very real, especially in the current climate of cost containment. Insurance claims and profiles of employees who generate a disproportionate share of health insurance costs are becoming available to managers in employee benefits departments and to financial officers. Employees worry legitimately about how their jobs and careers could suffer were information released concerning emotional instability or use of alcohol or drugs. Working with a patient's employer should be considered only in the context of confidentiality of the physician-patient relationship. The most important lesson is that there should never be a reason to reveal information to a patient's employer without first obtaining the patient's express consent.

Acknowledgments. This chapter is based on research funded in part by grants from The Commonwealth Fund, The National Institute on Alcohol Abuse and Alcoholism, and the Pew Memorial Trust.

References

1. Trice HM, Roman PM: *Spirits and Demons at Work*. New York, Cornell University Press, 1972.
2. Erfurt JC, Foote A: *Occupational Employee Assistance Programs for Substance Abuse and Mental Health Problems*. Ann Arbor, Worker Health Program, Institute of Labor and Industrial Relations, University of Michigan and Wayne State University, 1977.
3. Wrich JT: *Guidelines for Developing an Employee Assistance Program*. New York, American Management Assoc, 1982.
4. Egdahl RH, Walsh DC, Goldbeck WB: *Mental Wellness Programs for Employees*. New York, Springer-Verlag, 1980.
5. Walsh DC: Employee assistance programs. *Milbank Mem Fund Q/Health Soc.* 1982;60:492–517.
6. US Department of Health, Education and Welfare, Public Health Service, National Institute on Alcohol Abuse and Alcoholism: *Fourth Special Report on Alcohol and Health*. Government Printing Office, 1981.
7. US Department of Health and Human Services, Public Health Service, National Institute on Alcohol Abuse and Alcoholism: *Fifth Special Report on Alcohol and Health*. Government Printing Office, 1984.
8. Saxe L: *The Effectiveness and Costs of Alcoholism Treatment*. Health Technology Case Study 22. Congress of the United States, Offices of Technology Assessment, 1983.
9. Kurtz NR, Googins B, Howard WC: Measuring the success of occupational alcohol programs. *J Stud Alcohol* 1984;45:33–45.
10. Walsh DC, Hingson RW: Where to refer employees for treatment of drinking problems: The limited evidence from empirical research. *J Occup Med* 1985;27(10): 745–751.
11. Walsh DC: Is there a doctor in house? *Harvard Business Rev* July-August, 1984; 162(4):84–94.

References

[illegible]

Part V
Pathophysiology and Medical Complications

Every physician is familiar with the myriad of diseases resulting from chronic alcohol use and abuse. Well-recognized diseases, such as Wernicke's encephalopathy and alcoholic cardiomyopathy, are familiar to nearly every medical student. Less well known are the wide-ranging effects of alcohol on other disorders, such as hypertension, oral and esophageal cancer, and bowel motility. This section reviews a variety of diseases with one common denominator—they are caused or significantly affected by alcohol. These chapters are intended to be as clinically relevant as possible and aim to summarize both the major clinical syndromes and more subtle findings associated with alcoholism and alcohol abuse.

13
The Nervous System

JUDYANN BIGBY

Chronic alcohol use, whether excessive or moderate, can have major effects on both the central and peripheral nervous systems. Some of the complications are dependent on concurrent nutritional deficiencies, but in some cases, the role of nutritional deficiency is speculative or unclear.

Wernicke-Korsakoff Syndrome

Wernicke-Korsakoff syndrome is caused by thiamine (vitamin B_1) deficiency. Alcoholism is commonly associated with thiamine deficiency due to a combination of inadequate intake of vitamin B_1 and inhibition by alcohol of gastrointestinal transport of thiamine. Even in severe alcoholism, the syndrome will not develop if thiamine intake is adequate. In chronic liver disease, the capacity of the liver to store thiamine is decreased, as is change to the active form.

Based on autopsy studies, it is estimated that 12% of alcoholics suffer from Wernicke's encephalopathy, although the disease is often unrecognized before death, probably because of its variable clinical manifestations. The prevalence of thiamine deficiency is higher than 12%, suggesting that factors other than thiamine deficiency are important in the pathogenesis. Some data suggest that genetic factors may be important.[1,2]

Wernicke's encephalopathy and Korsakoff's psychosis have been described as two separate syndromes, Wernicke's encephalopathy as the acute onset of the classic triad of ocular abnormalities, ataxia, and global confusion, and Korsakoff's syndrome as anterograde and retrograde amnesia due to chronic, untreated thiamine deficiency. In a group of 186 patients with Wernicke's encephalopathy, Victor et al[3] demonstrated that 80% developed Korsakoff's syndrome. Other studies suggest that Wernicke's encephalopathy is more likely to be a chronic, relapsing illness and that patients rarely have the classic triad of symptoms. Data from pathologic examinations exist to support the hypothesis that the lesions leading to Wernicke's encephalopathy develop insidiously or during recurrent episodes of severe thiamine deficiency.[4] Therefore, Wernicke-

Korsakoff syndrome is best described as ocular abnormalities, ataxia, confusion, and amnesia occurring in various combinations.

Bilateral lateral gaze nystagmus is the most common ocular abnormality, followed by bilateral paralysis of the lateral rectus muscle. Other ocular manifestations include sluggish pupillary responses, anisocoria, ptosis, retinal hemorrhage, and papilledema. The ataxia in Wernicke's encephalopathy is similar to that described in alcoholic cerebellar degeneration. Patients have a wide-based stance and gait and, in severe cases, may not be able to walk. Ataxia of the trunk is also common. The upper extremities are usually not affected. Nystagmus, dysarthria, tremors, and other signs of cerebellar disease are rare. Vestibular paresis also contributes to the disequilibrium. Global confusion is a manifestation of acute Wernicke's encephalopathy, but there also may be generalized cognitive impairment, inattention, and memory deficit. Korsakoff's syndrome is manifest by anterograde amnesia (inability to learn new facts) and retrograde amnesia (inability to recall events from the past). Confabulation is not a classic or consistent feature of Korsakoff's psychosis.[2,5,6]

Acute Wernicke's encephalopathy is a medical emergency, since patients can progress to coma if left untreated. Mortality has been reported as high as 20% in some case series, but most patients had comorbid diseases, such as pneumonia and cirrhosis. Treatment with thiamine results in improvement in the ocular symptoms within one to six hours. If the lateral rectus palsy, ptosis, or vertical gaze paresis persists for more than one to two weeks after treatment, an etiology other than thiamine deficiency should be considered, although the vertical gaze nystagmus may persist for months. Improvement of the symptoms of cerebellar degeneration is less complete. Recovery may be expected in 40% of patients in one to four weeks after the initiation of treatment. Rapid recovery from the acute confusional state can be expected with thiamine treatment, but apathy and drowsiness may persist for longer periods. Often the memory deficits associated with Korsakoff's syndrome are apparent only after patients recover from the confusional states seen in acute Wernicke's encephalopathy. Only about 25% of alcoholic patients with mental status abnormalities due to Korsakoff's syndrome will recover with thiamine replacement. Nearly all patients with pure thiamine deficiency, such as that seen in malnourished prisoners of war, will recover when thiamine is replaced. Therefore, alcohol itself probably plays a role in the development of cognitive impairment in patients with alcoholism and thiamine deficiency.[5,6]

In acute Wernicke's encephalopathy with ocular findings, parenteral thiamine should be given in 100 mg increments up to 1000 mg or until the ocular abnormalities are reversed. Thiamine may be replaced in 100 mg increments orally, intravenously, or intramuscularly every day for five days. Since thiamine is a cofactor in glucose metabolism, glucose administration can precipitate or exacerbate acute Wernicke's encephalopathy, and thiamine should be given before any glucose. In addition, resistance to thiamine may result from hypomagnesemia due to magnesium's role as a cofactor for thiamine transketolase.[6] Magnesium sulfate should be given to all alcoholics with suspected acute Wernicke's encephalopathy, since most alcoholics have some degree of hypomagnesemia.

Peripheral Neuropathy

Polyneuropathy may result from deficiency of B-complex vitamins (thiamine, pyridoxine, and pantothenic acid) in combination with excess alcohol use. The pathologic changes are similar to those seen in diabetic peripheral neuropathy. The exact prevalence among alcoholics is unknown, since a substantial number may be asymptomatic despite abnormal neurophysiologic testing. The onset of symptoms is insidious, with a slowly progressive course. The typical symptoms are pain, paresthesias, and weakness. The lower extremities are usually affected alone, but concurrent upper extremity involvement may occur in approximately 30% of patients. Patients complain of pain in the distal portion of the lower extremities that progresses proximally without treatment. The pain may be described as a dull ache, as sharp and lancinating, as tightness in the muscles, or as cramps. The paresthesias can be a particularly distressing burning sensation, often precipitated or exacerbated by light tactile stimuli, such as sheets or clothing. The paresthesias are generally in the glove-stocking distribution. In severe cases, motor involvement leads to atrophy and weakness of the distal muscle groups. The autonomic nervous system may be involved, as evidenced by impotence, postural hypotension, and bowel or bladder dysfunction.[6,7]

On physical examination, patients have loss or diminution of the deep tendon reflexes, especially at the Achilles tendon. Sensory examination reveals loss of superficial touch and vibratory and position sense. Motor weakness and atrophy of distal muscle groups may be present and are usually symmetric. Only about one third of patients demonstrate involvement of deep tendon reflexes and motor and sensory systems simultaneously. The remaining two thirds may have one or two modalities involved.[8] Other signs that may be present include postural hypotension and excessive sweating of the soles of the feet or volar surfaces of the hands. The diagnosis is usually made on a clinical basis; confirmatory evidence includes slowed nerve conduction velocity and denervation of muscles as demonstrated by electromyography.

Replacement of the B-complex vitamins and abstinence from alcohol are the only forms of treatment. Physical therapy should be offered to patients with motor involvement to prevent deterioration and contractures. Improvement, which is incomplete in most cases, may take as long as five to six months once abstinence has been achieved.[9] It is unclear what role other agents, such as phenytoin, carbamazepine, and antidepressants (frequently used to treat diabetic peripheral neuropathy), have in treating the symptoms of alcoholic polyneuropathy. Patients with severe paresthesias may benefit from blocks of the lumbar sympathetic ganglia.

Syndromes Possibly Related to Nutritional Deficiency

Tobacco-alcohol amblyopia occurs primarily in undernourished alcoholics. It is unclear what role the excessive use of alcohol and tobacco plays in the onset of the disease, although observation of prisoners during World War II and the Korean conflict suggest that inadequate nutrition is the most important factor. The diagnosis is made on clinical grounds. Alcoholics complain of gradually progressive blurring and dimness of vision. Bilateral central scotomata are demonstrated on physical examination. The fundi are normal. B-complex vitamin replacement may reverse the condition.[6]

Other, rarer conditions believed to be secondary to alcoholism and poor nutrition are central pontine myelinolysis and Marchiafava-Bignami disease. There have been approximately 100 cases of central pontine myelinolysis reported. This condition is characterized by progressive quadriparesis, pseudobulbar palsy, and partial or complete paralysis of horizontal eye movements. Pathologically, it is characterized by selective demyelination of the corpus callosum. Marchiafava-Bignami disease is characterized by dysarthria, aphasia, frontal release signs, gait disturbances, urinary incontinence, increased motor tone, confusion, and hallucinations. At autopsy, there is symmetrical degeneration of myelin and axons in the central portion of the corpus callosum. Histologically, the abnormalities resemble those in central pontine myelinolysis. The exact etiology of these syndromes is uncertain, and no specific treatment is known.[4,6]

Alcoholic Cerebellar Degeneration

Alcoholic cerebellar degeneration is characterized by truncal ataxia and a wide-based stance and gait. The upper extremities are less affected than the lower. The progression of symptoms is slow but may be exacerbated by acute intoxication, metabolic abnormalities, or alcohol withdrawal.

The exact cause of alcoholic cerebellar degeneration is unknown, but there is growing evidence that it is not an entity separate from the cerebellar disease associated with Wernicke-Korsakoff syndrome.[4] Histologically, the changes in patients with alcoholic cerebellar degeneration are identical to those seen in Wernicke's encephalopathy. Cerebellar degeneration has been described also in patients with pure thiamine deficiency without alcoholism, and thiamine treatment reverses the syndrome. It appears that nutritional deficiencies play a role in the development of alcoholic cerebellar degeneration, and it may occur with other symptoms or as the only symptom of Wernicke-Korsakoff syndrome.[4]

The diagnosis is made on clinical grounds, although in some cases computerized tomography may demonstrate cerebellar atrophy. Abstinence from alcohol and nutritional treatment may result in improvement in 40% to 60% of the patients over several months.[4,6]

Alcoholic Dementia

Cognitive impairment is one of the most common neurologic complications of chronic alcoholism. In studies of the etiology of dementia, alcoholism accounts for 6% to 21% of cases. Defects in new learning, visual spatial function, abstract thinking, and psychomotor skills can be demonstrated to some degree in all chronic drinkers, including early-stage alcoholics and social drinkers.[10] Malnutrition may play a role in the development of intellectual impairment, but there is evidence that alcohol or its metabolites cause brain dysfunction. The degree of impairment corresponds to the chronicity of drinking. Clinically, patients with alcoholic dementia show memory deficits and global intellectual deterioration. Clinical studies have suggested that patients with gradual onset of Korsakoff's psychosis are similar to patients with alcoholic dementia—there is higher prevalence among females, it occurs at an early age, and patients improve or do not progress if they abstain from alcohol.[11] There is probably some overlap of the two syndromes.

Computerized tomography has demonstrated cerebral atrophy in alcoholics of all ages at a higher rate than in nondrinking controls, but this finding is not consistent and is probably influenced by nutritional factors and age. It is unclear whether the degree of cerebral atrophy corresponds with the degree of cerebral dysfunction, since strong concordance between neuropsychologic testing and atrophy has not been demonstrated. In one study, cerebral atrophy reversed with abstinence.[12] There have been no consistent pathologic changes found in patients with alcoholic dementia or atrophy associated with excess alcohol use. Abstinence from alcohol is the only known treatment, and patients can be expected to improve somewhat or (at the very least) show no progression in the impairment. It is important for physicians to recognize that most alcoholics will have some degree of cognitive impairment, and interviewing and treatment strategies should take this into account.

Alcohol-Withdrawal Seizures

Withdrawal seizures occur in 4% to 16% of alcoholics withdrawing from alcohol. Ninety percent occur within 48 hours of abstaining or decreasing alcohol consumption. Most occur in 24 hours, but they can occur as late as seven days after stopping drinking. The seizures are usually grand mal, and 60% of the patients have two or more seizures. Status epilepticus is rare. One third of untreated patients who have withdrawal seizures progress to delirium tremens.[13]

Patients with new seizures should be evaluated with computerized tomography and EEG, since alcoholic patients may suffer from multiple episodes of head trauma, with resultant structural seizure foci. In addition, withdrawal from alcohol makes an individual more susceptible to seizures caused by other factors, making a history of recent withdrawal from alcohol less useful in determining the cause. The EEG reflects the effect of alcohol on the brain: abnormal during intoxication, returning to normal with cessation of drinking, periods of dysrhythmia during early abstinence, and then returning to normal. Except during the period of early abstinence, the prevalence of abnormalities in the EEG in patients with alcohol withdrawal seizures does not differ from that of normal individuals. Treatment of alcohol withdrawal seizures is described in Chapter 10.

Hepatic Encephalopathy

Hepatic encephalopathy occurs with severe liver failure of any cause and is, therefore, a common complication of excessive alcohol use due either to acute alcoholic hepatitis or to cirrhosis with portal–systemic shunting. The exact cause of hepatic encephalopathy is not known but is probably secondary to the failure of the liver to detoxify substances, such as ammonia or gamma-aminobutyric acid (GABA), derived from the intestine. Ammonia is generated by the action of bacteria on nitrogenous substances and is normally metabolized in the liver. In the presence of liver disease or portal–systemic shunting, ammonia enters the systemic circulation and crosses the blood-brain barrier. In the brain, it is converted to glutamine. Ammonia is known to cause coma in animals and is a likely cause of the abnormalities seen in hepatic encephalopathy. GABA is produced in the intestinal tract by bacterial action on protein and metabolized by the liver. Patients with hepatic failure have high GABA-like activity in their serum, and increased concentrations of GABA in animals can induce coma and contribute to neuroinhibition. Receptor sites for GABA in the brain are associated closely with receptors for benzodiazepines and are increased in animals with hepatic failure.

Other toxins that have been implicated in the etiology of hepatic encephalopathy are mercaptans, short-chain and medium-chain fatty acids, and phenol. The encephalopathy is probably secondary to a group of toxins that act synergistically to increase cerebral sensitivity to physiologic and pharmacologic derangements.[14,15]

Early signs of hepatic encephalopathy are subtle and nonspecific. They include inappropriate behavior, mood swings, including agitation, depression, and apathy, and change in sleep habits. At this time, asterixis may not be present, and the diagnosis may be difficult to make. Formal mental status testing will be abnormal but nonspecific. Confusion, disorientation, a depressed mental status, and coma develop if early hepatic encephalopathy is left untreated, and asterixis is present at this stage. Other abnormal physical findings that help make the diagnosis are presence of fetor hepaticus (a characteristic sweetish odor of the patient's breath), neurologic signs, such as tremor, rigidity, or hyperreflexia, and signs of chronic liver disease and portal–systemic shunting, such as palmar erythema or spider angiomata. Laboratory results useful in making the diagnosis are abnormal liver function tests, hypoalbuminemia, and, in particular, a prolonged prothrombin time. The EEG is usually abnormal and reveals symmetrical, high-voltage, slow wave patterns. The arterial level of ammonia is usually abnormal but may be normal and does not correlate with the degree of encephalopathy. The level of glutamine in the cerebral spinal fluid is elevated. Other causes of metabolic encephalopathy should be ruled out before a diagnosis is made.

Hepatic encephalopathy is reversible in most patients, although the mortality rate is extremely high once a patient has developed coma. Common precipitants of encephalopathy in patients with underlying liver disease are renal insufficiency with an increase in blood urea nitrogen, electrolyte abnormalities, gastrointestinal bleeding, excess dietary protein, infection, and constipation. Most of these conditions cause an increase in the production of ammonia or other toxins, or they alter the blood- brain barrier, causing enhanced diffusion of toxins into the brain. Patients are particularly susceptible to sedatives and tranquilizers, perhaps due to the increased number of receptors in the brain.

Treatment of hepatic encephalopathy usually results in improvement of mental status in 24 to 48 hours. Any underlying conditions should be treated. The main goal of therapy is to reduce the amount of protein in the intestinal tract, thereby decreasing the amount of toxin production. Dietary protein should be restricted and reintroduced into the diet in 20 g increments. Chronically, patients should restrict dietary protein to 30 to 40 g/day. Neomycin reduces the number of colonic bacteria, thereby decreasing the production of ammonia and other toxins and should be given in doses of 2 to 12 g/day depending on the degree of compromise. Laxatives should be given to evacuate intestinal contents. Lactulose, a synthetic disaccharide that acidifies bowel contents and thereby reduces back diffusion of ammonia, can be given chronically in a dose to achieve three to four loose bowel movements each day. Hemoperfusion through charcoal may be useful for patients in coma unresponsive to other treatments.[16] Branch-chain amino acids have not proved effective in the treatment of hepatic encephalopathy.[17]

Discussion

Neurologic complications from drinking alcohol are common. Wernicke-Korsakoff syndrome should be viewed as a continuum of clinical problems rather than as two separate clinical syndromes. Cognitive impairment is the most common neurologic manifestation of alcoholism, but some degree of impairment has been demonstrated by neuropsychologic testing in social drinkers as well. Cognitive dysfunction, manifested by poor memory and inconsistencies in the medical history, may interfere with the physician's ability to obtain reliable historical data when evaluating patients and when following them through treatment. Since cognitive impairment improves with abstinence, physicians should reiterate the reasons for abstaining and the treatment goals once the patient has stopped drinking in order to increase the patient's understanding of his underlying disorder and increase the prospect for compliance.

References

1. Lishman WA: Cerebral disorder in alcoholism: Syndromes of impairment. *Brain* 1981;104:1-20.
2. Thomson AD: Alcohol-related structural brain changes. *Br Med J* 1982;38:87-91.
3. Victor M, Adams RD, Collins GH: *The Wernicke- Korsakoff Syndrome*. Philadelphia, FA Davis, 1971.
4. Harper C: Neuropathology of brain damage caused by alcohol. *Med J Aust* 1982;2:277-282.
5. Reuler JB, Girard DE, Cooney TG: Wernicke's encephalopathy. *N Engl J Med* 1985;312:1035-1039.
6. Nakada T, Knight RT: Alcohol and the central nervous system. *Med Clin North Am* 1984;68:121-131.
7. Victor M: Polyneuropathy due to nutritional deficiency and alcoholism, in Dyke PJ, Thomas PK, Lambert EH (eds). *Peripheral neuropathy*. Philadelphia, WB Saunders, 1975, pp 1030-1066.
8. Behse F, Bachthal F: Alcoholic neuropathy: Clinical and electrophysiological and biopsy findings. *Ann Neurol* 1977;2:95-110.
9. Hawley RJ, Kurtzke JF, Armbrustmacher VW, et al: The course of alcoholic-nutritional peripheral neuropathy. *Acta Neurol Scand* 1982;66:582-589.
10. Parker DA, Parker ES, Brody JA, et al: Alcohol use and cognitive loss among employed men and women. *Am J Public Health* 1983;73:521-526.
11. Parker ES, Noble EP: Alcohol consumption and cognitive functioning in social drinkers. *J Stud Alcohol* 1977;33:1224-1232.
12. Carlen PL, Wortzum G, Holgate C, et al: Reversible cerebral atrophy in recently abstinent chronic alcoholics measured by computed tomography scans. *Science* 1978;200:1076-1078.
13. Thompson WC: Management of alcohol-withdrawal syndromes. *Arch Intern Med* 1978;138:278-283.
14. Ferenci P, Schafer DF, Kleinberger G, et al: Serum levels of gamma-aminobutyric acid in acute and chronic hepatocellular disease. *Lancet* 1983;2:811-813.
15. Schafer DF, Jones EA: Hepatic encephalopathy and the gamma-aminobutyric acid neurotransmitter system. *Lancet* 1982;1:18-20.
16. Gunson AES, Brande S, Mellin PS, et al: Earlier charcoal hemoperfusion in fulminant hepatic failure. *Lancet* 1982;2:681-683.
17. Warren J, Denis J, Desurmont P, et al: Is intravenous administration of branch chain amino acids effective in treatment of hepatic encephalopathy? A multicenter study. *Hepatology* 1983;3/4:475-480.

14
The Liver

ANNE W. MOULTON and MICHELE G. CYR

Alcoholic liver disease is the most common and perhaps most devastating medical consequence of chronic alcohol abuse. Because alcohol is metabolized primarily in the liver, its toxic effects are concentrated there, producing fatty liver, hepatitis, and cirrhosis. The relationship between alcohol and cancer of the liver is discussed in Chapter 18.

Epidemiology

The association between alcohol abuse and hepatic diseases has been known for centuries. Although a minority of alcoholics develop cirrhosis (8% to 30% according to studies of liver biopsies and autopsies), a high percentage of cirrhotics have underlying alcoholism if they live in areas where per capita consumption of alcohol is high. The prevalence of alcoholism among cirrhotics ranges from 66% to 42% in the Americas and Europe to a low of 11% in Asia.[1,2] In the United States, mortality from alcoholic cirrhosis accounts for 50% of the 35,000 cirrhosis-related deaths annually.[3] In 1981, it was the second leading cause of death in New York City for people aged 25 to 44. Alcoholism and alcoholic liver disease are increasing in both younger and female populations.

The incidence of serious liver disease increases as a function of both quantity and duration of alcohol use, with considerable individual variation. There may be additional factors that modify alcohol's effect on the liver. Hepatic steatosis or fatty liver may develop after moderate consumption of 20 to 40 g/day of absolute alcohol (1½ to 3 drinks/day). In contrast, alcoholic hepatitis occurs only after drinking for an extended period. Studies from France and Germany suggest that 160 to 180 g/day of alcohol consumed for ten to 25 years represents the average dose associated with progression to cirrhosis. Yet, risk of cirrhosis is increased significantly with even moderate daily consumption of alcohol (40 g for males and 20 g for females).[4]

The amount of alcohol consumption required for the development of cirrhosis in females is 50% that for males, and some of this discrepancy can be attributed to the difference in lean body weight. In addition to differences in size, women have a greater proportion of adipose tissue (33%) than men (25%), which results in higher serum concentrations of alcohol. Women alcoholics appear at greater risk for developing cirrhosis, progressing to that stage after shorter periods of alcohol consumption (13 years versus 20 years in one study).[5]

The binge drinker is at less risk than the steady drinker, presumably because the liver has time to regenerate between bouts of heavy drinking. This finding may reflect lower total consumption of alcohol in binge drinkers. There is no established relationship between type of alcoholic beverage consumed and severity of alcoholic liver disease.

Metabolic Effects

Ethanol is metabolized primarily in the liver (90% to 98%). Because of alcohol's affinity for hepatic enzyme systems, it displaces up to 90% of other substrates normally used in the liver. Ethanol is metabolized primarily via alcohol dehydrogenase to acetaldehyde and hydrogen, which is transferred to nicotinamide-adenine dinucleotide (NAD). The change in the NADH:NAD ratio causes many of the metabolic abnormalities associated with alcoholic liver disease, including increased fatty acid accumulation, hyperlacticacidemia and secondary hyperuricemia, and hypoglycemia.

Metabolism of acetaldehyde proceeds via the same pathway as ethanol, generating NADH and probably enhancing its own toxicity in the liver. Acetaldehyde plays an important role in hepatic steatosis, causing hepatomegaly secondary to the swelling of hepatocytes with proteins as well as lipids. In addition to depressing hepatic mitochondrial function, acetaldehyde interacts with a variety of substances within the liver, producing hepatotoxic effects that may have a further role in the pathogenesis of alcoholic liver disease.

Prolonged exposure to high doses of alcohol induces increased activity of the microsomal ethanol oxidizing system (cytochrome P-450) in the liver. Enhanced activity in this system accelerates clearance of alcohol and production of acetaldehyde and other toxic products, and potentiates the hepatotoxic effects of drugs metabolized in the liver, for example, acetaminophen and isoniazid. However, this enzyme induction does not contribute significantly to the development of tolerance, which is primarily a phenomenon of central nervous system adaptation.

Additional Factors

Several additional factors in the development of alcoholic liver disease have been studied to explain varying susceptibility to alcohol- induced injury. These include nutritional deficiencies, increased genetic susceptibility, associated viral hepatitis, alterations of the immune system, and female gender.

Early work suggested that malnutrition might play a primary role in alcoholic liver disease (especially hepatitis and cirrhosis). Subsequent animal studies have disproved this hypothesis, but the role of malnutrition in the promotion of toxic effects of alcohol needs further clarification.[1] The role of genetics in the toxicity of alcohol has been investigated (earlier, kindred studies and, more recently, studies looking at specific traits, eg., HLA), but these studies have not produced any consistent associations.

Although hepatitis B may occur with increased frequency in certain populations of alcoholics, there is no convincing evidence to date that previous hepatitis B infection plays a role in progression to cirrhosis among chronic alcoholics. In contrast, recent studies suggest that previous hepatitis B may have a role in the development of hepatocellular carcinoma in alcoholic cirrhosis.[6]

There are several lines of evidence to suggest that altered immunity may perpetuate damage done to the liver by alcohol: serum from patients with alcoholic hepatitis or cirrhosis suppresses lymphocyte transformation, antibodies to Mallory bodies have been identified; and serum immunoglobulins (especially IgA) are elevated in alcoholics. It has not been established whether these changes are primary or secondary phenomena. The suggestion that altered immunity may play a larger role in the development of alcoholic liver disease in women has not been widely accepted.

Spectrum of Alcoholic Liver Disease

There is considerable overlap in both pathology and clinical presentation among the three stages of liver disease.

Hepatic Steatosis (Fatty Liver)

Fat accumulation in the liver is the earliest effect of alcohol, and it can occur with even modest consumption of alcohol (20 to 40 g/day) in normal drinkers.[7] It is the most common abnormality found on liver biopsy in chronic alcoholics, occurring in up to 90%. Because of the mechanisms discussed previously, fatty acids are deposited in the liver, initially within the cytoplasm of hepatocytes and eventually in globules, usually located near the central hepatic vein. Steatosis is graded from 0 to 4+, depending on the percentage of liver cells that contain fat (under 25% = 1+; over 75% = 4+). Changes in the ultrastructure of mitochondria and smooth endoplasmic reticulum are also observed (as in alcoholic hepatitis). Hepatic steatosis is thought not to progress to cirrhosis, but up to 40% of patients with fatty liver will have pericentral fibrosis without evidence of diffuse alcoholic hepatitis.[1] This fibrosis may lead to postsinusoidal portal hypertension and ascites before the development of cirrhosis.

Patients with fatty liver may have no symptoms[7] or complain of right upper quadrant tenderness, nausea, vomiting, and anorexia.[2] Seventy-five percent of patients have hepatomegaly, but a much smaller percentage have jaundice or ascites. Complications, including severe cholestasis, portal hypertension, and esophageal varices, are rare. Laboratory data may be normal or include moderately elevated transaminases or a slightly elevated alkaline phosphatase or bilirubin.[1,7,8]

In more severe cases, alcoholic steatosis may mimic alcoholic hepatitis, and a liver biopsy may be helpful for diagnosis. Steatosis may also coexist with hepatitis and cirrhosis. Alone, fatty liver is thought to be a benign disease, and with abstinence, resolution of symptoms should occur in two weeks and histology revert to normal in four to six weeks. In chronic alcoholics who continue to drink, fatty liver progresses to alcoholic hepatitis in a substantial proportion of cases.

Alcoholic Hepatitis

Alcoholic hepatitis is a clinical syndrome with well-established histologic criteria but variable presentation, ranging from no symptoms to florid hepatic failure. It occurs after chronic, excessive consumption of alcohol and may be either acute or chronic, frequently coexisting with fatty liver or cirrhosis.

The histology of alcoholic hepatitis is characterized by four types of change: hepatocellular necrosis (swollen hepatocytes and cellular debris), inflammatory exudate (mononuclear and polymorphonuclear cells), fibrosis and sclerosis, and the accumulation of cytoplasmic glycoproteins called alcoholic hyalin or Mallory bodies.

Patients may be asymptomatic with alcoholic hepatitis or ill with anorexia and weight loss, nausea and vomiting, abdominal pain, and fever and chills.[7,9] They demonstrate hepatomegaly in 80% to 98% of cases and less often have jaundice (35% to 80%), ascites (25% to 75%), and spider angiomata (20% to 70%).[9]

Laboratory data may reveal an elevated bilirubin (usually mild to moderate), elevated transaminases with aspartate aminotransferase (AST) in the range of 100 to 500 and an AST:ALT (alanine aminotransferase) ratio of 2 to 5:1, and significant elevations of alkaline phosphatase, suggesting cholestasis. Serum proteins are frequently depressed, but serum globulins are frequently elevated. Prothrombin time is often prolonged. Anemia, thrombocytopenia and leukopenia are common, as is leukocytosis which correlates well with the severity of the hepatitis. Ultrasound is a relatively insensitive screen for alcoholic hepatitis. Liver-spleen scans are a little more sensitive and add information about hepatic dysfunction.

The role of liver biopsy in the management of alcoholic hepatitis is controversial. Because there is a substantial overlap clinically among the different stages of liver disease, a liver biopsy is the only way to make a definitive diagnosis. A liver biopsy may be useful in cases where the history suggests more than one possible etiology for liver disease, for example, in drinking patients with positive hepatitis B serologies or an elevated serum iron. Clearly, the liver biopsy should not replace taking an extensive drinking history. Twenty percent of patients in one case series of chronic alcoholics with suspected alcoholic liver disease had other diagnoses that mimicked alcoholic liver disease and were potentially treatable.[10] However, repeated liver biopsies in chronic alcoholics with frequent admissions to the hospital for hepatitis are not warranted.

The prognosis for patients with alcoholic hepatitis is difficult to determine. Prognostic studies based on liver biopsy are biased by patient selection (asymptomatic patients or severely ill patients with ascites and coagulopathy are often excluded)[8] and by the subjective nature of biopsy interpretation. Furthermore, the variable relationship between the structural changes and the clinical status of the patient and the coexistence of other liver disease limit the usefulness of these studies. More accurate predictors of prognosis may be physiologic measures of liver function, such as prothrombin time, bilirubin, or albumin, or the clinical status, especially the presence of ascites. Finally, the major determinant of outcome for the chronic alcoholic with acute hepatitis is not histology but cessation of alcohol consumption.

Therapy for alcoholic hepatitis is primarily supportive. Treatment should include correction of fluid and electrolyte imbalance as well as deficiencies in phosphorus, magnesium, and vitamins, including folic acid, thiamine, and iron. No therapy to date has been shown to affect substantially either the short-term prognosis of alcoholic hepatitis or the progression to cirrhosis. Studies using corticosteroids or anabolic steroids in patients with severe alcoholic hepatitis have produced conflicting results.[11] Therapies without clear benefit that have been investigated include insulin and glucagon, propylthiouracil, D-penicillamine, and colchicine.

Most patients with alcoholic hepatitis have a mild course, although a significant percentage (10% to 15%) have a prolonged course or die. Factors that predict decreased survival in alcoholic hepatitis include prolonged prothrombin time, elevated serum bilirubin concentration, the presence of encephalopathy, progressive renal failure, and severity of the histologic lesions.[11] Estimates for overall mortality from alcoholic hepatitis do not take into account the more benign cases of hepatitis that often go undetected. Most patients recover in six weeks to six months with abstinence. After recovery, histology may show total resolution, residual pericentral or perisinusoidal fibrosis, chronic hepatitis, or progression to micronodular cirrhosis. As many as 50% of patients with alcoholic hepatitis who continue to drink will develop cirrhosis.

Laennec's (Micronodular) Cirrhosis

Cirrhosis develops in a moderate percentage of chronic alcoholics (8% to 30%).[1,2] This has led to speculation about the role alcohol plays—the amount, the duration, and other factors. It is difficult to separate quantity and extent of alcohol abuse to determine their relative contributions, since the amount of alcohol consumption increases with the duration of alcohol abuse. Studies suggest that consumption of more than 160 g/day (200 ml of ethanol, one pint of whiskey, for 15 years) is the critical dose-duration factor in the development of cirrhosis.[2]

Laennec's cirrhosis is distinguished histologically by fibrosis and regeneration. Increased collagen synthesis is a major factor in the development of cirrhosis, but it is unknown whether this is a direct effect of alcohol, a reaction to hepatic inflammation and necrosis, or secondary to an immunologic mechanism. Decreased collagen breakdown also may play a role. Normal architecture is distorted by scarring (bands of tissue separate lobules into smaller islands of cells) and is disrupted further by regenerating nodules. As a result, the normal lobular architecture is replaced by pseudolobules that lack a portal space or efferent venous channels. These changes are directly responsible for the subsequent portal hypertension and hepatocellular dysfunction in cirrhosis. Other markers of alcoholic liver disease may be present, including fat droplets, large mitochondria, Mallory bodies, and perivenular and perisinusoidal fibrosis. Iron deposits are especially common in alcoholic cirrhotic livers.

Signs and symptoms show considerable overlap with other stages of alcoholic liver disease and may include failure to thrive (anorexia, weight loss, weakness, and fatigability), jaundice, low-grade fever, and abdominal discomfort. Complaints of upper abdominal pain may relate to concurrent reflux esophagitis, gastritis, peptic ulcer disease, acute hepatitis, or gallstones. Specific symptoms relating to hepatic dysfunction or portal hypertension include hepatic encephalopathy, ascites, splenomegaly, esophageal varices, and hemorrhoids. In addition, patients may demonstrate parotid enlargement, spider angiomata, palmar erythema, Dupuytren's contractures, and signs of secondary endocrine dysfunction, including gynecomastia, testicular atrophy, amenorrhea, or impotence.

Laboratory studies are nonspecific. Transaminases are only moderately elevated, with a ratio of AST:ALT of greater than two. Other liver function tests are variably elevated. Additional abnormalities, which depend on the degree of cirrhosis and complications, include low serum albumin, potassium, phosphorus, and magnesium, abnormal clotting studies with deficiencies in clotting factors, and thrombocytopenia. Ultrasound can identify diffuse parenchymal disease but cannot differentiate cirrhosis from fatty liver reliably. The liver-spleen scan and CT scan are equally accurate in the detection of diffuse hepatocellular disease, although the former appears to be more sensitive in the detection of cirrhosis. The liver biopsy is very sensitive in cirrhosis, subject to only a 5% sampling error, which is increased in the presence of macronodular cirrhosis.[8,12]

Complications of alcoholic cirrhosis are multiple: the sequelae of varices and variceal bleeding, ascites, portal hypertension, hepatorenal syndrome, spontaneous bacterial peritonitis, portasystemic encephalopathy, and hepatoma. The development of ascites is the most common sequela of chronic cirrhosis. In addition to portal hypertension, decreased serum albumin and renal retention of sodium and water contribute to ascites formation. The treatment of uncomplicated ascites should include removal of any medications that inhibit prostaglandin synthesis, bedrest if possible, dietary restriction to a 2 gram sodium diet with fluid restriction to 2 L/day, and treatment with spironolactone. Maximum diuresis of ascitic fluid should not exceed 1 L/day. Approximately 5% of patients will not respond to conservative treatment and will require the insertion of a Leveen peritoneovenous shunt.

Bleeding from esophageal varices is a major cause of mortality for patients with alcoholic cirrhosis. Immediate mortality is 60% to 70% during an acute episode, and there is substantial risk of rebleeding and death within the next two weeks. Optimum 5-year survival rates of approximately 59% are noted after placement of selective distal splenorenal shunt.[11] Sclerotherapy appears to reduce acute bleeding but may have less effect on survival.[12] Studies using propranolol to prevent recurrent bleeding have produced conflicting results. Acutely, placement of the portasystemic shunts has a high perioperative mortality. If performed electively, the placement of a shunt may prevent rebleeding and prolong survival in some patients.[11]

The mortality from cirrhosis is significant, and prognosis is also affected by the factors listed for hepatitis. Cessation of drinking appears to lessen the risk of death in all patients except those with severe cirrhosis, portal hypertension, and varices. One study suggested a five-year survival of only 40.5% of patients who continue to drink but 63% of those who stopped drinking. These patients were divided into subgroups based on complications of ascites, jaundice, and hematemesis, and five-year survival rates were as follows: patients who had none of the three complications and who stopped drinking had a survival rate of 88.9% in contrast to 68.2% in those who continued to drink. Patients who had one or more of the three complications and stopped drinking had a survival rate of 60.1% in contrast to the five-year survival rate of 34% in those who continued drinking.[13]

The literature suggests that some cirrhotics will attempt to cut down or stop drinking when confronted with the diagnosis (21% to 35% of the patients in five studies).[14] At the other end of the spectrum are the 50% to 80% of patients who survive a life-threatening complication of alcoholic liver disease and return to drinking, in some cases heavily (20% to 50%).[13] Additional studies examining the impact of medical complications on the natural history of chronic alcoholism will clarify the role of medical intervention. Treatment of alcoholic liver disease has changed little in the last 20 years. The most important role for the general internist is to convince the alcoholic patient with liver disease to stop drinking.

References

1. Lieber CS, Leo MA: Alcohol and the liver, in Lieber CS (ed): *Medical Disorders of Alcoholism: Pathogenesis and Treatment.* Philadelphia, WB Saunders, 1982, pp 259–312.
2. Pimstone NR, French SW: Alcoholic liver disease. *Med Clin North Am* 1984;68: 39–56.
3. Burnett DA, Sorrell MF: Alcoholic cirrhosis. *Clin Gastroenterol* 1981;10:443–455.
4. Tuyns AJ, Pequinot G: Greater risk of ascitic cirrhosis in females in relation to alcohol consumption. *Int J Epidemiol* 1984;13:53–57.

5. Saunders JB, Davis M, Williams R: Do women develop alcoholic liver disease more readily than men? *Br Med J* 1981;282:1140–1143.
6. Brechot C,Nalpas B, Courouce AM, et al: Evidence that hepatitis B virus has a role in liver-cell carcinoma in alcoholic liver disease. *N Engl J Med* 1982;306:1384–1386.
7. Bruguera M, Bordas JM, Rodes J: Asymptomatic liver disease in alcoholics. *Arch Pathol Lab Med* 1977;101:644–647.
8. Rankin JGD, Orreggo-Matte H, Deschenes J, et al: Alcoholic liver disease: The problem of diagnosis. *Alcoholism Clin Exp Res* 1978;2:327–338.
9. Fallon HJ: Alcoholic hepatitis, in Schiff L, Schiff ER (eds): *Diseases of the Liver*, ed 5. Philadelphia, JB Lippincott, 1982, pp 39–56.
10. Levin DM, Baker AL, Riddell RH, et al: Nonalcoholic liver disease: Overlooked causes of liver injury in patients with heavy alcohol consumption. *Am J Med* 1979;66:429–434.
11. Galambos JT: Alcoholic liver disease: Fatty liver, hepatitis, and cirrhosis, in Berk JE (ed): *Gastroenterology*. Philadelphia, WB Saunders, 1985, 2985–3048.
12. Cello JP, Grendell JH, Crass RA, et al: Endoscopic sclerotherapy versus portacaval shunt in patients with severe cirrhosis and acute variceal hemorrhage: Long-term follow-up. *N Engl J Med* 1987;316(1):11–15.
13. Schenker S: Alcoholic liver disease: Evaluation of natural history and prognostic factors. *Hepatology* 1984;4:36S–43S.
14. Hermos JA: Drinking by alcoholic cirrhotic patients under medical care: A literature survey. *Alcoholism Clin Exp Res* 1984;8:314–318.

15
The Gastrointestinal Tract and Pancreas

MICHELE G. CYR and ANNE W. MOULTON

Alcohol has pervasive effects on the gastrointestinal tract and pancreas, ranging from subtle microscopic changes to devastating clinical sequelae. As the portal of entry into the body, the digestive tract is vulnerable to the effects of alcohol. The effect of alcohol on the pancreas is mediated by less direct mechanisms. The association between alcohol and liver disease is discussed in Chapter 14 and that with gastrointestinal cancer is discussed in Chapter 18.

Oropharynx and Salivary Glands

Despite repeated exposure of the oral cavity to high concentrations of alcohol, changes directly attributable to alcohol are few. Instead, nutritional deficiencies are primarily responsible for the stomatitis, glossitis, and cheilitis of chronic alcoholics and are easily reversible with the institution of an adequate diet.[1,2] Parotid glandular enlargement is present in approximately 50% of alcoholics with chronic liver disease but is much less common in those without coexistent hepatic dysfunction.[1] Alcohol does, however, decrease the quantity and increase the viscosity of saliva, which impairs the normal buffering and flushing action of saliva on the esophagus and may contribute to the pathogenesis of alcohol-induced esophagitis.[3] The clinical significance of glossitis, stomatitis, cheilitis, and parotid enlargement lies primarily in their role as markers for underlying nutritional deficiencies and liver disease.

Esophagus

Both acute and chronic alcohol ingestion are associated with functional abnormalities of the esophagus. Acute exposure to alcohol produces consistent alterations in esophageal motility. Lower esophageal sphincter pressure is decreased, impairing the most potent antireflux mechanism of the esophagus, and peristalsis is generally depressed.[3,4] Deranged esophageal motility is frequently observed in alcoholics who have autonomic neuropathy. In these patients, esophageal primary peristaltic waves (propulsive) are reduced, and tertiary peristaltic waves (nonpropulsive) are increased, resulting in defective esophageal clearance.[1,3] These alterations are more a manifestation of the associated autonomic neuropathy than a direct effect of chronic alcohol exposure.

Alcohol also exerts damaging effects on the esophageal mucosa, mainly by enhancing hydrogen ion penetration into mucosal cells, causing histologic changes of inflammation. In the absence of $H+$ ions, the direct toxic effects of alcohol have been questioned, but the presence of acid clearly augments any direct effects.[3]

The clinical consequences of alcohol abuse follow logically from the observed alterations of normal esophageal function. Impaired lower esophageal sphincter function increases the likelihood of gastroesophageal reflux, accounting for the frequent complaint of heartburn among drinkers. This greater propensity for acid reflux, coupled with defective clearance, predisposes alcoholics to acute and chronic esophagitis, peptic stricture, and Barrett's esophagus.[2,5] Frequently, the esophagitis resolves with abstinence alone, but conventional antireflux regimens may enhance healing.

Esophagitis, esophageal varices, and Mallory-Weiss tears can all cause hematemesis. Studies indicate that up to 40% of patients with Mallory-Weiss lesions are alcoholic.[3] Contrary to earlier suspicions, gastroesophageal reflux does not increase the likelihood of hemorrhage from esophageal varices in patients with cirrhosis and portal hypertension.[1]

Stomach

Alcohol's effect on gastric motility is directly related to the concentration of alcohol in the gastric fluid. At low concentrations, the effect is variable; at high concentrations, gastric emptying is uniformly delayed.[2] Delayed gastric emptying is caused by the suppression of motor function and not by the induction of pylorospasm.[1]

Conflicting evidence exists about the effect of alcohol on gastric acid secretion.[4] The deleterious effects of alcohol on the gastric mucosa are caused by disruption of the gastric mucosal barrier, which permits back-diffusion of hydrogen ions into mucosal cells and produces the mucosal changes of acute gastritis: erythema, edema, exudates, and petechiae.[6] The role of alcohol in the development of chronic gastritis of the superficial and atrophic types remains controversial.[1,7] Although increased prevalence of chronic gastritis is observed among alcoholics, the relative contributions of alcohol exposure, nutritional deficiencies, and liver disease are not fully known.[8]

Acute gastritis is a frequent consequence of excessive alcohol ingestion. This has been confirmed endoscopically in subjects after a brief drinking binge.[4] Patients may have symptoms of anorexia, vomiting, and epigastric pain. Hemorrhagic gastritis may ensue from severe alcohol damage, especially with concurrent use of aspirin.[4] Although spontaneous cessation of bleeding is usual with abstinence, treatment with antacids or H_2 blocking agents is nonetheless warranted to minimize irritation to the injured mucosa. Symptoms of acute gastritis typically resolve within hours or, at most, two days.[8] The reversibility of chronic gastritis and the tendency for acute hemorrhage in this setting is controversial. Some evidence suggests that the chronically exposed gastric mucosa develops tolerance to the acute injurious effects of alcohol. Other evidence supports an increased susceptibility to alcohol-induced protein loss and hemorrhage.[4-9]

There is no clearly established relationship between alcohol consumption and the development of peptic ulcer disease, delayed ulcer healing, or higher treatment relapse rates. Associated factors, such as smoking, cirrhosis, portal hypertension, and pancreatitis, may predispose the alcoholic to peptic ulceration.[6]

The chronic alcoholic with upper gastrointestinal bleeding presents a challenging clinical problem. The variety of potential sources of bleeding often requires endoscopy to ensure appropriate diagnosis and therapy. Acute gastric mucosal lesions account for the majority of upper gastrointestinal bleeding events in chronic alcoholics (42.9% in one series), with a much smaller contribution from esophageal varices, esophagitis, Mallory-Weiss tears, peptic ulcer disease, or duodenitis.[1,8] Endoscopic studies have demonstrated that even when esophageal varices are present, they are the source of gastrointestinal bleeding in only 50% of cases.[1] Despite the predominance of acute gastric mucosal lesions as the cause of gastrointestinal bleeding in alcoholics, early endoscopy should be performed in patients suspected or known to have esophageal varices in order that specific therapy (pitressin, sclerotherapy, Sengstaken-Blakemore tube) can be instituted if variceal bleeding is confirmed.

Small Intestine

The action of alcohol on small bowel motility contributes to the diarrhea so frequently associated with both binge and chronic drinkers. Although alcohol has complex actions on small bowel motor function, its overall effect is to shorten intestinal transit time.[1,10,11]

Microscopic changes are most prominent in the duodenal and jejunal villi and ileal crypts after acute exposure to alcohol.[2] Chronic exposure leads to generalized derangements of villous architecture, with decreased villous height and reduced numbers of mucosal surface cells.[2,11] Both acute and chronic alcohol ingestion cause reversible disruption of the intestinal brush border enzyme systems, with depression of disaccharidase activity. Of particular clinical importance is lactase deficiency, which can cause significant lactose intolerance in binge and chronic drinkers.[1,2,11]

The principal functions of the small intestine, specialized transport and absorption, are altered by both acute and chronic alcohol ingestion. Disruption of active transport may account for the impaired absorption of water, sodium, glucose, and amino acids associated with alcohol ingestion.[2,7,11] Malabsorption of folate, vitamin B_{12}, thiamine, and calcium is also common and somewhat better understood. Folate deficiency, the most common nutritional deficiency of the alcoholic, is observed in 20% to 50% of chronic alcoholics.[12] Alcohol interferes with folate absorption, and the resultant folate deficiency causes small bowel morphologic and functional changes that compound the malabsorption of folate and other nutrients.[7,11] Vitamin B_{12} absorption is impaired through decreased secretion of intrinsic factor (IF) and abnormal binding of the IF–B_{12} complex to terminal ileal receptors.[2] Although vitamin B_{12} deficiency is relatively uncommon in alcoholics (10% in one series), the Schilling test is compatible with malabsorption.[7,11] Thiamine absorption is affected in the setting of reduced dietary intake when active transport is the predominant mechanism of absorption.[2] Calcium absorption is affected directly by alcohol's interference with duodenal transport and affected indirectly when abnormal vitamin D metabolism ensues from concurrent alcoholic liver disease.[1,7]

Thus, alcohol-induced alterations of normal intestinal motility, structure, and function contribute to the important problems of diarrhea, malabsorption, and malnutrition of the alcoholic. Rapid intestinal transit time, lactose intolerance, and impaired water and electrolyte absorption account for the frequent occurrence of diarrhea in both binge and chronic drinkers.[2-4] Steatorrhea can be documented in one third to one half of alcoholics.[1,11] Subclinical pancreatic exocrine insufficiency and abnormal hepatic bile salt excretion may impair intraluminal digestion and result in steatorrhea. This is usually reversible with abstinence unless associated with chronic irreversible disease of the pancreas or liver.[11] The malnutrition of the alcoholic is, therefore, not a simple matter of dietary insufficiencies but, rather, a consequence of the complex interactions of decreased intake, increased requirements, and impaired absorption.

Colon and Rectum

The colon and rectum are relatively spared from the effects of alcohol. Experimentally, acute administration of alcohol causes increased colonic propulsive activity, but the clinical importance of this is unclear.[1] Although rectal hemorrhoids are associated with cirrhosis and portal hypertension, significant bleeding is uncommon. Varices of the colon are similarly associated with cirrhosis and can cause massive rectal hemorrhage.[1]

Pancreas

With the exception of liver disease, pancreatitis is the most commonly recognized disease resulting from alcohol abuse. The incidence of alcoholic pancreatitis varies widely among countries and even within given populations, a variation that is largely a function of differences in alcohol consumption.[13,14] Chronic pancreatitis from all causes has a prevalence of 1 to 10/100,000, and an estimated 70% to 90% of cases in the United States are attributable to alcohol abuse.[15] Whereas only 5% to 10% of alcoholics have clinically apparent pancreatitis, as many as 40% to 50% may have pathologic evidence of disease.[5]

Both the absolute quantity of alcohol ingested and the duration of abuse are important factors in the development of pancreatic disease. With heavy consumption, clinical manifestations can become evident in from five to 15 years.[16] Additional contributing or permissive factors for the development of pancreatitis include nutritional status, genetic influences, and metabolic factors.[13]

The pancreatitis associated with alcohol is not pathologically distinct from that of other causes. Acute pancreatitis in its mild form is characterized by interstitial edema and inflammation and in its severe form by hemorrhage and necrosis. Chronic pancreatitis is marked by irreversible and frequently progressive changes of fibrosis, acinar cell destruction, duct dilatation, and calcification. The pathologic changes of acute pancreatitis are frequently superimposed on those of chronic pancreatitis.

Despite the clear epidemiologic link between alcohol and pancreatitis, the actual mechanism of injury remains elusive. Pancreatitis of any type is ultimately an inflammatory process resulting from autodigestion by pancreatic enzymes. One current hypothesis suggests that alcohol causes pancreatitis by the precipitation of protein plugs, with subsequent obstruction of the small peripheral pancreatic ducts.[17] Critics of this theory argue that the protein plugs are a secondary phenomenon and propose a direct toxic effect of alcohol or one of its metabolites on pancreatic cells.[14]

Acute pancreatitis is characterized by severe, poorly localized upper abdominal pain with radiation to the back, associated with nausea and vomiting, which is partially relieved by leaning forward. The pain may be precipitated by a drinking binge or a large meal. Physical examination may reveal low-grade or moderate fever, with tachycardia and relatively mild abdominal tenderness, given the severity of pain. No single laboratory test confirms the diagnosis, but the serum amylase remains the initial test of choice for the diagnosis of acute pancreatitis. Elevation of amylase 1.5 to 2 times the upper limit of normal has a sensitivity of 94.8% and specificity of 98.4% for the diagnosis of acute pancreatitis.[18] The proposed superior diagnostic accuracy of the amylase:creatinine clearance ratio remains controversial and only marginally increases the sensitivity compared to serum amylase alone. In the acute attack, serum lipase remains elevated longer than serum amylase and may be useful in suspected cases of pancreatitis with normoamylasemia.[13] Conversely, hyperamylasemia of salivary origin is present in a significant percentage of acutely intoxicated patients without pancreatitis.[14] The serum lipase, radioimmunoassay to trypsinogen, and the pancreatic isoamylase assay are equally useful tests for patients with hyperamylasemia to either confirm or exclude the diagnosis of acute pancreatitis.[18] Although pancreatic calcifications on plain abdominal x-ray strongly suggest the diagnosis of chronic alcoholic pancreatitis, they are not pathognomonic.[14] It is imperative that diagnostic tests for pancreatitis be interpreted within the context of the clinical presentation.

Management of mild cases of acute pancreatitis is directed toward limiting the inflammatory process and controlling pain. Oral feedings are withheld to prevent pancreatic secretion of enzymes. Nasogastric suction confers no added therapeutic benefit in the absence of vomiting or abdominal distention.[5] In most cases, narcotic analgesics are required to control pain.

In 80% to 90% of cases, conservative management leads to resolution of the acute attack within two to four days.[16] More severe cases may be complicated by hypotension and shock, renal failure, coagulopathy, pleuropulmonary abnormalities, metabolic instability, ascites, or pancreatic abscess or pseudocyst. Predictors of poor outcome have been well established by Ranson[5] and are elaborated in standard medical texts. Intensive medical support is required, and in cases of pancreatic abscess or pseudocyst, surgery may be necessary. Mortality for severe cases may be as high as 30%.[14]

Although chronic pancreatitis is often associated with severe abdominal pain, as many as 40% of patients are completely pain free.[15] The pain occurs either as distinct episodes of acute pancreatitis or as insidiously intensifying upper abdominal discomfort. Some patients may also have prominent symptoms relating to pancreatic exocrine and endocrine insufficiencies. Malabsorption occurs in up to 75% of patients with disease of eight to ten years' duration.[15] Diabetes is seen in one third of patients with pancreatic calcification, and an additional one third have abnormal glucose tolerance tests.[19] Other complications include biliary obstruction, pseudocyst formation, and upper gastrointestinal bleeding.

Management of chronic pancreatitis centers around pain control and treatment of complications. Abstinence from alcohol may diminish the pain but probably does not halt the progression of the disease toward the associated exocrine and endocrine insufficiencies. Although pain control poses a difficult management problem, surgical management appears no more efficacious than conservative treatment.[14] Steatorrhea is improved with enzyme replacement and reduction of dietary fat. Although the diabetes associated with pancreatic insufficiency is frequently mild, it may be difficult to control. Glucagon deficiency may be responsible for this erratic response to treatment.[14] Mortality from chronic pancreatitis is estimated at 3% to 4% per year, and approximately 40% to 50% of deaths in patients with chronic pancreatitis are directly attributable to the pancreatic disease and its complications.[19]

References

1. Lieber CS, Klingenstein J, Rubin DK: Alcohol and the digestive tract, in Lieber CS (ed): *Medical Disorders of Alcoholism: Pathogenesis and Treatment*. Philadelphia, WB Saunders, 1982, pp 363–411.
2. VanThiel DH, Lipsitz HD, Porter LE, et al: Gastrointestinal and hepatic manifestations of chronic alcoholism. *Gastroenterology* 1981;81:594–615.
3. Wienbech M, Wilhelm B: Esophageal lesions in the alcoholic. *Clin Gastroenterol* 1981;10(2):375–388.

4. Burbige EJ, Lewis DR Jr, Halstead CH: Alcohol and the gastrointestinal tract. *Med Clin North Am* 1984;68(1):77–89.
5. Ranson JHC: Acute pancreatitis: Pathogenesis, outcome, and treatment. *Clin Gastroenterol* 1984;13(3):843–863.
6. Domschke S, Domschke W: Gastroduodenal damage due to drugs, alcohol, and smoking. *Clin Gastroenterol* 1984;13(2):405–437.
7. Thomson AD, Majumdar SK: The influence of ethanol on intestinal absorption and utilization of nutrients. *Clin Gastroenterol* 1981;10(2):263–293.
8. Valencia-Parparcen J: Alcoholic gastritis. *Clin Gastroenterol* 1981;10(2):389–399.
9. Geokas MC, Lieber CS, French S, Halstead CH: Ethanol, the liver, and gastrointestinal tract. *Ann Intern Med* 1981;95:198–211.
10. Belk IT, Dinda PK: Acute exposure of small intestine to ethanol: Effects on morphology and function. *Dig Dis Sci* 1981;26(9):817–838.
11. Green HR: Alcohol, nutrition, and malabsorption. *Clin Gastroenterol* 1983;12(2):563–575.
12. Longman MJS, Bell GD: Alcohol and the gastrointestinal tract. *Br Med Bull* 1982;38(1):71–75.
13. Pirola RC, Lieber CS: Acute and chronic pancreatitis, in Kissin B, Begleiter H (eds): *The Biology of Alcoholism*. New York, Plenum Press, 1978, vol 3, *Clinical Pathology*.
14. Lieber CS, Korsten MA, Pirola RC: Alcoholic pancreatitis: Experimental and clinical features, in Lieber CS (ed): *Medical Disorders of Alcoholism: Pathogenesis and Treatment*. Philadelphia, WB Saunders, 1982, pp 412–435.
15. Worning GH: Chronic pancreatitis: Pathogenesis, natural history and conservative treatment. *Clin Gastroenterol* 1984;13(3):871–894.
16. Geokas MC: Ethanol and the pancreas. *Med Clin North Am* 1984;68(1):57–75.
17. Sarles H, Laugier R: Alcoholic pancreatitis. *Clin Gastroenterol* 1981;10(2):401–414.
18. Steinberg WM, Goldstein SG, Davis ND, et al: Diagnostic assays in acute pancreatitis: A study of sensitivity and specificity. *Ann Intern Med* 1985;102:576–580.
19. Lake Bakaar G: Alcohol and the pancreas. *Br Med Bull* 1982;38(1):57–62.

16
Nutritional Status, Cardiovascular, Hematologic, Reproductive, and Musculoskeletal Systems

JACK ENDE

The range of medical complications from alcohol consumption extends across almost every organ system, touching on numerous bodily functions. This chapter emphasizes the relationship between alcohol and illness as the primary care physician encounters it.

Nutrition

Alcoholism is a major cause of malnutrition in the Western world. Diseases that should be relegated to the pages of outdated textbooks can still be found, albeit rarely, in populations suffering from alcoholism. Nutritional problems are most prevalent among skid row alcoholics, but more affluent heavy drinkers are not spared.

Alcohol impairs nutrition in a variety of ways.[1] Alcohol substitutes for food in the diet, but its calories are metabolically inferior to those of normal foodstuff. In addition, alcohol suppresses the appetite both centrally and as a result of gastritis, and it damages the organs of digestion—the liver, the pancreas, and the small intestine. Finally, it interferes with metabolism and activation of other dietary constituents.

The consequences of alcohol-induced nutritional deficiencies are variable, and physical examination may not show evidence of malnutrition. There is always the concern that the manifestations of important nutritional deficiencies may be delayed by several years or be so subtle that they are not detected by routine clinical assessment. When there are symptoms and signs of malnutrition, they tend to be nonspecific. Weight loss and feelings of fatigue, lassitude, and weakness can be found in most cases of alcohol-induced protein-calorie malnutrition. Such patients are also likely to have signs of multiple vitamin deficiencies. Findings common to many vitamin deficiencies, such as a wasted appearance, flaking skin, sparse thin hair, glossitis and cheilosis, edema, and abdominal distention, may be present. In advanced cases, specific syndromes may be identified. Alcoholics, especially those with cirrhosis, are prone to deficiencies of B vitamins, niacin, ascorbic acid, and folate.[2]

Thiamine deficiency can cause neurologic disease (dry beriberi) and cardiac disease (wet beriberi). Most patients have involvement of both systems, although occasionally dysfunction of one or the other system will predominate. The neurologic findings of thiamine deficiency include peripheral neuropathy with paresthesias, muscle pain, and weakness and the Wernicke-Korsakoff syndrome (Chapter 13). The cardiac complications of thiamine deficiency are the result abnormal peripheral vasodilatation that occurs in these patients for reasons that are unclear. As vascular resistance falls, cardiac output rises. Indeed, cardiac output may become so elevated that vascular congestion, edema, and transudative effusions are found. Interestingly, treatment with thiamine often results in a period of systemic hypertension as the arteriovenous channels close while cardiac output is still high. Beriberi heart disease occurs far less commonly than alcoholic cardiomyopathy due to the toxic effects of alcohol on the heart muscle. In contrast to beriberi heart disease, the cardiac output is low in alcoholic cardiomyopathy and the peripheral resistance is secondarily high. The neurologic and cardiac sequelae of thiamine deficiency should be treated with parenteral thiamine, 50 mg daily, until the patient can resume a normal diet. Oral thiamine supplements will prevent recurrent deficiency.

Riboflavin deficiency results in cheilosis, stomatitis, seborrheic dermatitis, and conjunctivitis. Additional ocular findings include photophobia, lacrimation, and corneal neovascularization. The diagnosis can be confirmed if there is decreased 24-hour urinary excretion of riboflavin.

Alcoholics are at increased risk for pyridoxine deficiency because ethanol interferes with the metabolism of pyridoxal-5-phosphate, the active form of the vitamin. The risk of pyridoxine deficiency is increased by certain drugs, such as isoniazid and penicillamine. The clinical expression of pyridoxine deficiency is variable but includes sideroblastic anemia and neuritis. Suspected cases should be treated with pharmacologic doses, 50 to 100 mg, of pyridoxine daily.

Niacin deficiency, or pellagra, begins characteristically as a generalized mucositis involving the tongue, mouth, gastrointestinal tract, and, in women, the vagina. This explains the diarrhea, the first of the three Ds of pellagra. Pellagra also causes dermatitis and dementia. The skin involvement is a photosensitivity reaction, which, in the early stages, may be indistinguishable from sunburn. It progresses to hyperpigmentation and thickening of the sun-exposed areas, followed by similar changes in areas of chronic irritation, such as the axilla, groin, and under the breasts in women. The intellectual changes of pellagra are nonspecific. Severely affected patients may be disoriented or frankly psychotic. Patients respond to supplemental niacin.

Vitamin C deficiency, or scurvy, occurs with increased frequency in alcoholics. Early symptoms include lassitude, irritability, and generalized aches and pains. Diagnosis is evident from the characteristic changes in the skin: perifollicular hyperkeratotic papules, especially on the posterior thighs. The hairs within these follicles coil inward and become buried, and the perifollicular zones become hemorrhagic. Generalized bleeding into the skin and soft tissue is present in advanced scurvy. Gums are swollen, spongy, friable, and bleed easily. Reduced plasma levels of vitamin C are diagnostic. In suspected cases, therapy should not be withheld until the diagnosis is confirmed. Vitamin C, 100 mg four times per day by mouth, should be started without delay.

Although patients with identifiable deficiencies are interesting, such patients are not encountered frequently in general practice. Far more common is the alcoholic patient who has nonspecific signs of vitamin or protein–calorie malnutrition or who has no evidence of nutritional deficiency at all. Optimal management for all alcoholic patients, with and without clinical stigmata, includes a well-balanced diet, discontinuation of drinking, and multivitamin therapy, in addition to correction of any specific deficiencies that are identified. Appropriate resources should be recruited to ensure adequate meals for patients who continue to drink heavily and who are unable to manage for themselves.

Fetal Effects

Maternal alcohol abuse affects fertility adversely and increases the risk of spontaneous abortion.[3] When pregnancy is carried to term, the infant has an increased risk of congenital anomalies. These vary from mild intrauterine growth retardation to the fetal alcohol syndrome.[4]

The fetal alcohol syndrome, or fetal alcohol effect, is evident in one third or more of children born to severely alcoholic women who consume six or more drinks per day. The complete syndrome is a disorder with diverse manifestations. These infants have reduced body weight and height, and they may have central nervous system dysfunction, typically attention-deficit disorders, hyperactivity, or mental retardation. Their facies may be recognizable by a cluster of abnormalities: short palpebral fissures, midfacial hypoplasia, short, upturned noses, absence of the ridge between the nose and upper lip, and a thin upper lip. The phenotypic expression of the syndrome varies from infant to infant, but as a group, these children leave little doubt of alcohol's harmful effects on fetal development.

The most vulnerable period for alcohol-induced injury to the fetus is early in the first trimester. This means that the maldevelopment arising from heavy drinking may occur before the woman realizes she is pregnant. Alcoholic women of childbearing age should be told about the risks of birth defects if they become pregnant and continue to drink. Recommendations for light-drinking or moderate-drinking mothers are more controversial. Epidemiologic studies suggest that women who drink more than one drink per day give birth to slightly smaller infants. Such results must be interpreted with caution, however, because of the confounding influences of malnutrition, smoking, and drug use, each of which can affect fetal growth. Since no safe level of alcohol intake has been established, pregnant women should be advised to keep alcohol consumption to a minimum or, better still, abstain entirely.

Cardiac Disease

Alcohol is capable of affecting the cardiovascular system in many ways and may influence the manifestations of heart disease from other etiologies. The association between alcohol and heart failure does not depend on malnutrition. The cardiomyopathy of thiamine deficiency (wet beriberi) is encountered primarily in the disadvantaged, skid row alcoholic. The well-nourished alcoholic patient develops heart disease related directly to the biochemical and ultrastructural effects of alcohol. The clinical picture of alcohol cardiomyopathy is nonspecific. Symptoms and signs of biventricular failure, an enlarged cardiac silhouette on x-ray, and an abnormal ECG offer little to distinguish alcoholic cardiomyopathy from other causes of heart disease. Stigmata of alcoholism may be present, but many patients with severe alcoholic heart disease have minimal involvement of other organ systems.

The diagnosis of alcoholic cardiomyopathy is based on the alcohol history: heavy drinking in excess of ten years is the rule. Because other forms of heart disease begin later in life, alcoholic cardiomyopathy should be considered as a diagnosis for heart failure in patients under the age of 50. The disease begins with a preclinical phase of varying duration during which the patient is asymptomatic, but noninvasive tests reveal significant dysfunction. Chamber enlargement is detected by echocardiography and systolic-time intervals show decreased contractility. Arrhythmias occur during this phase, particularly after heavy binges. The so-called holiday heart syndrome,[5] typically occurring after weekends or holidays, refers to atrial fibrillation, atrial flutter, premature ventricular beats, or other evidence of cardiac irritability that disappears without residual effect in a person without clinical evidence of heart disease.

If the patient continues to drink, chronic symptoms develop. Patients have fatigue, decreased exercise tolerance, or symptoms of arrhythmia. At this stage, the myocardial changes that have occurred are still considered reversible. Once the clinical features of congestive cardiomyopathy appear, the damage is likely to be permanent. Abstinence is associated with longer survival, but in many patients, the disease progresses even after the patient stops drinking. Therefore, early diagnosis and prevention are of utmost importance.

There is considerable interest in the effects of alcohol on coronary artery disease. Alcohol intake at moderate levels is associated with a decreased incidence of atherosclerosis and a reduced risk of myocardial infarction.[6] High density lipoprotein (HDL) cholesterol levels in plasma are elevated in moderate drinkers, and originally, the benefit of alcohol on atherosclerosis was thought to be on that basis. However, the particular HDL subfraction elevated by moderate alcohol intake is HDL-3, whereas epidemiologic data have associated HDL-2 with reduced incidence of coronary artery disease.[7] The mechanism for alcohol's protective effect remains unclear.

There is a question of safety in the use of alcohol for the patient with established coronary artery disease. Alcohol in small amounts (two and five ounces) has been shown to raise the pulse and systolic blood pressure, decrease the duration of exercise required to produce angina pectoris, and accentuate the ST depression that occurs with exercise.[8] The importance of these findings has not been established. At present, it seems most prudent to advise patients with coronary artery disease to limit alcohol consumption and, if they do drink, not to do so before exercising.

Alcohol affects the metabolism and threshold for toxicity of medications commonly used in the cardiac patient. Warfarin is metabolized by the microsomal ethanol oxidizing system and is degraded more rapidly in the abstaining patient who habitually consumes large amounts of alcohol. Yet it is metabolized more slowly in that same patient if he is drinking. The net effect is unpredictable levels of anticoagulation. Heavy drinkers are frequently deficient in potassium and magnesium and are, therefore, prone to digitalis toxicity.

Hypertension

Numerous epidemiologic studies have found an association between hypertension and moderate-to-heavy alcohol consumption.[9,10] The association is strongest for middle-aged, white men who consume more than three drinks per day. In this group, a ten mm increase in systolic pressure and a smaller, though significant, increase in diastolic pressure can be demonstrated. Excess alcohol consumption also appears to interfere with the efficacy of therapy. Heavy drinkers are overrepresented in population studies that identify patients whose hypertension is difficult to control with standard medical therapy. Cohort studies support the association between alcohol and blood pressure. Alcoholic hypertensives have been found to become normotensive with abstinence and to become hypertensive again if they resume drinking. A recent prospective study suggested that alcohol may have a direct pressor effect, although the mechanism remains elusive.[11] Reduction in alcohol consumption appears to have a favorable effect on blood pressure control in treated hypertensives.[12]

The Joint National Committee on Detection, Evaluation and Treatment of High Blood Pressure recommended that, to control hypertension, patients who drink should do so moderately (ie, less than 60 g/day of alcohol, equivalent to less than four ounces of 100 proof whiskey, eight ounces of wine, or 24 ounces of beer).[13] Undoubtedly there are large differences in how an individual hypertensive patient responds to alcohol or to abstinence, but the effect of alcohol on blood pressure appears to be of practical importance. Alcohol should always be kept in mind as a remediable factor that may be contributing to a patient's hypertension or interfering with treatment.

Hematology

The hematologic consequences of alcohol come from nutritional deficiencies and liver disease and directly from alcohol's toxic effect on the bone marrow.[14] The characteristic morphologic change in the bone marrow of patients who drink heavily is vacuolization of the primitive cells, especially proerythroblasts. Although this change is nonspecific and disappears within weeks of abstaining, it can be a useful sign of heavy drinking.

Even more useful is the finding of macrocytosis on the peripheral blood smear. An elevated MCV, in the absence of anemia, should alert the clinician to the possibility of alcoholism. The morphologic abnormality is typically mild (MCVs in the 100 to 115 range). In contrast to the macroovalocytosis of folate deficiency, the cells are round, not oval shaped, and the granulocytes are not hypersegmented. After heavy drinking ceases, the macrocytosis of alcoholism persists for weeks, sometimes up to two months. When present, this finding can be helpful in identifying the heavily drinking patient and in monitoring abstinence, although it lacks sufficient sensitivity to be a useful screening test for alcoholism. The mechanism for the macrocytosis of alcoholism is obscure.

Anemia in the alcoholic can be hemorrhagic, hemolytic, or hypoplastic, and, of course, more than one mechanism can operate in a given patient.[15] Bleeding can result from the gastrointestinal complications of alcoholism or coagulation defects. The hemolytic anemias found in alcoholic patients are a consequence of liver disease and portal hypertension, compounded by alcohol's marrow-suppressive effect. They arise from alterations of the red cell membrane due to the lipoprotein abnormalities of liver disease and from hypersplenism. The most common membrane alteration, the formation of target cells, is not associated with anemia; indeed, target cells are more resistant to extravascular destruction. The clinical point, therefore, is that finding target cells on the peripheral smear in an anemic patient does not explain the anemia.

When hemolytic anemia is present, it is usually mild (hematocrit usually 30% or greater), with spherocytes found on peripheral smear. A more severe hemolytic anemia, characterized by spur cells, is found in certain patients with far advanced cirrhosis and portal hypertension. Hematocrits here are less than 30%, sometimes as low as 15%, and reticulocytosis is in the 5% to 15% range. Normal red cells, when transfused into patients with spur cell anemia, become similarly affected.

Hypoplastic anemia in the alcoholic can be due to bone marrow suppression or folate deficiency. Folate deficiency is common among alcoholics because of poor nutrition and direct interference by alcohol with folate absorption and activity. The diagnosis of folate deficiency should be made from the peripheral smear. Typical are macroovalocytic red cells and hypersegmented neutrophils, the latter present even when there is a superimposed microcytic process. The bone marrow in folate deficiency shows typical megaloblastic changes. Measured serum levels and even erythrocyte folate levels may be falsely low due to alcohol ingestion. Therefore, folate levels are of limited value in the diagnostic workup of the alcoholic patient with anemia unless typical morphologic changes are present on peripheral smear. The anemia of folic acid deficiency responds promptly to dietary therapy: bone marrow changes may vanish in a day, and reticulocytosis follows within a week of therapy. Hypersegmented neutrophils may continue to provide evidence of folate deficiency for a week or two after other changes have receded. Vitamin B_{12} deficiency is not associated with alcoholic intake or with cirrhosis.

Another form of hypoplastic megaloblastic anemia in the alcoholic is sideroblastic anemia. These patients have anemia and elevated serum iron levels. The peripheral blood smear shows a dimorphic picture, with both macrocytic and hypochromic microcytic red cells. The bone marrow reveals characteristic ringed sideroblasts. Alcoholic sideroblastic anemia is often associated with pyridoxine deficiency. Treatment should include proper diet, pharmacologic doses of pyridoxine (100 mg/day), and abstinence from alcohol.

Leukopenia is found in about 3% of alcoholics admitted to the hospital.[16] This may arise from folate deficiency, hypersplenism, infection, or as a direct result of alcohol on the bone marrow. In the last case, there may or may not be concomitant depression of red cells and platelets. When leukopenia is associated with infection, recovery is often followed by a rebound leukocytosis. When due to bone marrow depression without infection, the reduced white count rises more sluggishly, usually reaching normal levels in one to two weeks after admission to the hospital and cessation of alcohol consumption. Alcohol has been associated with impairment of granulocyte function, diminished macrophage motility, and abnormalities in lymphocyte transformation.

Coagulation problems are common in cirrhosis due to diminished production of the vitamin K-dependent factors (VII, IX, X, and prothrombin) as well as fibrinolysis and disseminated intravascular coagulation.[17] Platelet counts may be low secondary to hypersplenism and folic acid deficiency and as a direct action of alcohol's decreasing platelet production and shortening platelet survival. The significance of alcohol-induced thrombocytopenia is variable and unpredictable. In some patients, thrombocytopenia contributes to clinically important hemorrhage. In others, the diminished platelet count proves of no consequence. No correlation is found between alcohol-induced thrombocytopenia and either anemia or leukopenia. In patients with thrombocytopenia related to alcohol, the platelet count begins to rise two or three days after drinking ceases and then reaches a peak (often transiently above normal) in a week or two.

Endocrinologic Disease

Alcohol affects gonadal function adversely at many levels. Toxicity to the testes, the pituitary, and the hypothalamus in men has been demonstrated repeatedly. In the male alcoholic, hypogonadism may be manifested by reduced beard growth, loss of libido and potency, and abnormal sperm analysis. Testicular atrophy is found in severe cases. All this can occur in the absence of liver disease. With the development of cirrhosis, feminization occurs, including gynecomastia and redistribution of body hair and fat.[18]

Impotence and loss of libido may be the problem that first makes the heavy drinker seek medical attention. Alcohol-induced hypogonadism should always be considered before embarking on an elaborate workup for impotence. In many cases, the prognosis is good. Unless testicular atrophy (defined as pole-to-pole measurement less than two and a half cm) is present, there is a good chance that the patients who stops drinking will regain normal sexual functioning within a few months.[19] Abstinent patients without testicular atrophy who continue to have erectile dysfunction months after cessation of alcohol require evaluation for other causes of impotence.

Alcohol influences a great many other endocrine systems. The posterior pituitary–hypophyseal system is inhibited by alcohol. Following ingestion of ethanol, vasopressin levels fall, accounting for the well-known diuretic effect of alcohol. Alcohol also accounts for a pseudo-Cushing's syndrome.[20] In part due to chronic alcoholism and in part due to cirrhosis, there is a subset of patients who develop moon facies, truncal obesity, buffalo humps, proximal muscle weakness, hypertension, and osteoporosis. These patients have biochemical evidence of Cushing's syndrome that remits within days or weeks after drinking is stopped. Metabolic effects of alcohol, including hypomagnesemia, hypocalcemia, hypoglycemia, and ketoacidosis, are discussed in Chapter 17.

Musculoskeletal Diseases

In the musculoskeletal system alcohol can cause acute and chronic myopathy and a number of bone problems. Acute alcoholic myopathy (also referred to as "alcoholic rhabdomyolysis") usually follows a bout of heavy drinking.[21] The diagnosis is most secure when there is no history of trauma. However, patients who have sustained trauma but who seem to have myositis out of proportion to their trauma fit this category as well. These patients have painful, tender, swollen muscles in one or more large groups. Symptoms persist for a few days and then resolve, with residual weakness lasting months. Muscle enzymes are markedly elevated and myoglobin may be present in the urine. During the acute phase, patients must be kept well hydrated and monitored carefully for acute tubular necrosis. When the affected muscles are in a closed compartment (the lower leg, for instance), a second wave of muscle necrosis may complicate the course if muscle swelling is so great that it compromises vascular supply. In such patients, fasciotomy may be required.

The pathogenesis of acute alcoholic myopathy is not known. At times, one encounters alcoholic patients who have no muscle tenderness but who manifest a rise in muscle enzymes within a few days of admission to the hospital. This subclinical form of alcoholic myopathy has been associated with hypophosphatemia and suggests that the acute fulminant syndrome may be a manifestation of hypophosphatemia as well. A more chronic form of alcoholic myopathy may accompany alcoholic polyneuropathy. This type of myopathy is painless, with progressive muscle weakness and wasting. It occurs in chronic alcoholics with coexistent nutritional deficiencies.

Alcohol is an important factor in the development of metabolic bone disease. Although the mechanism is not clear, drinking even in moderation is a risk factor for osteoporosis.[22] This is a concern particularly for slender, white women, with other risk factors for osteroporosis, however, men who drink heavily appear to be at risk for bone loss as well.[23] Postmenopausal women who drink should be considered for preventive therapy with calcium and, if appropriate, estrogen.

Osteonecrosis, or avascular necrosis of bone, has been associated with alcoholism in middle-aged men.[24] The disease occurs most commonly in the head of the femur, where it is bilateral in 50% of patients. Patients complain of hip pain and demonstrate limitation of motion without evidence of arthritis elsewhere. Plain radiographs may lag behind the clinical presentation but eventually will show patches of subchrondral lucency and increased density, representing areas of dead bone and areas of repair. The mechanism for this is obscure. Osteonecrosis may be due to fat emboli to bone from alcoholic fatty liver. Suspected patients should be hospitalized, treated with bedrest, and followed carefully. Bone grafts may be helpful. In severe cases, total hip prosthesis is indicated.

Miscellaneous Problems

Alcohol impairs the immune system and lowers resistance to infection.[25] The bactericidal activity of polymorphonuclear leukocytes is affected adversely by alcohol, as is the ability of the alveolear macrophage to cleanse the tracheobronchial tree. Matters are made worse by the alcoholic's tendency toward aspiration due to CNS depression and interference of the glottis closure during intoxication. Alcoholics are at increased risk for pulmonary infection, in particular gram-negative and anaerobic aspiration pneumonias and lung abscesses.[26] Tuberculosis is also associated with alcoholism.

A variety of dermatologic problems are related to alcoholism.[27] Some have already been discussed in the nutrition and endocrine sections of this chapter and in Chapter 14. The skin may also be affected directly as a result of the excessive use of alcohol. A common manifestation is the suffused, reddened face, especially the nose, and the edematous eyelids and injected conjunctivae considered tell-tale signs of alcoholism. These findings are suggestive of alcohol excess, but they should not be overinterpreted. Rosacea and rhinophyma, related conditions characterized by rose-red papules and nodules symmetrically distributed across the face and nose, are not caused by excessive drinking. Alcohol intensifies the appearance of rosacea and rhinophyma but does not bring on the lesions de novo. Porphyria cutanea tarda (PCT), characterized by photosensitivity and blistering skin lesions leading to scarring, is found with increased frequency among alcoholics with liver disease.[28] Facial hair growth is increased in PCT. Finally, alcoholics are more likely than similarly predisposed abstainers to manifest clinical hemochromatosis, including the diffuse bronze pigmentation of the skin.

Discussion

Alcohol in excess impacts on health in many ways, and few, if any, of these are beneficial. The primary care physician who is familiar with the medical complications of alcoholism will be able to anticipate problems and begin management in a timely fashion. Many problem drinkers have medical complications. Whether or not these patients suspect their symptoms are due to alcohol, they may deny the association. By convincing the patient that the medical problem and the alcohol problem are linked, the physician has a powerful tool that may lead the patient to therapy.

References

1. Morgan MY: Alcohol and nutrition. *Br Med Bull* 1982;38:21–29.
2. Leevy CM, Thomson AD, Baker H: Vitamins and liver injury. *Am J Clin Nutr* 1970;23:493–499.
3. Pratt OE: Alcohol and the developing fetus. *Br Med Bull* 1982;38:48–52.
4. Clarren SK, Smith DW: The fetal alcohol syndrome. *N Engl J Med* 1978;298:1063–1067.
5. Regan TJ, Haider B: Ethanol abuse and heart disease. *Circulation* 1981;64(III):14–19.
6. Devenyi P, Robinson GM, Roncari DAK: Alcohol and high-density lipoproteins. *Can Med Assoc J* 1980;123:981–984.
7. Haskell WL, Camargo C Jr, Williams PT, et al: The effect of cessation and resumption of moderate alcohol intake on serum high density lipoprotein subfractions: A controlled study. *N Engl J Med* 1984;310:805–810.
8. Orlando J, Aronow WS, Cassidy J, Prokash R: Effect of ethanol on angina pectoris. *Ann Intern Med* 1976;84:652–656.
9. Klatsky AL, Friedman GD, Siegelaub AB, Gerard MJ: Alcohol consumption and blood pressure: Kaiser-Permanente multiphasic health examination data. *N Engl J Med* 1977;296:1194–1200.
10. Wallace RB, Lynch CF, Pomrehn PR, et al: Alcohol and hypertension: Epidemiologic and experimental considerations. *Circulation* 1981;64(III):41–47.
11. Potter JF, Beevers DG: Pressor effect of alcohol in hypertension. *Lancet* 1984;2:119–122.
12. Puddey IB, Beilin LJ, Vandongen R: Regular alcohol use raises blood pressure in treated hypertensive subjects: A randomized controlled trial. *Lancet* 1987;1:647–651.
13. The Joint National Committee on Detection, Evaluation and Treatment of High Blood Pressure: The 1984 report of the Joint National Committee on detection, evaluation and treatment of high blood pressure. *Arch Intern Med* 1984;144:1045–1057.
14. Herbert V (ed): Hematologic complications of alcoholism. *Semin Hematol* 1980;17:83–176.
15. Chanarin I: Hemopoiesis and alcohol. *Br Med Bull* 1982;38:81–86.
16. Liu YK: Effects of alcohol on granulocytes and leukocytes. *Semin Hematol* 1980;17:130–136.
17. Cowan DH: Effect of alcoholism on hemostasis. *Semin Hematol* 1980;17:137–147.
18. Van Thiel DH: Ethyl alcohol and gonadal function. *Hosp Pract* 1984; November: 1952–1958.
19. Van Thiel DH, Gavaler JS, Sanghvi A: Recovery of sexual function in abstinent alcoholic men. *Gastroenterology* 1982;84:677–682.
20. Smals A, Kloppenborg P, Njo K, et al: Alcohol-induced cushingoid appearance. *Br Med J* 1976;2:1298.
21. Perkoff GT, Dioso MM, Bleisch V, et al: A spectrum of myopathy associated with alcoholism. I. Clinical and laboratory features. *Ann Intern Med* 1967;67:481–482.

22. Heaney RP, Gallagher MD, Johnston CC, et al: Calcium nutrition and bone health in the elderly. *Am J Clin Nutr* 1982;36:986–1013.
23. Spencer H, Rubio N, Rubio E, et al: Chronic alcoholism: A frequently overlooked cause of osteroporosis in men. *Am J Med* 1986;80:393–397.
24. Saville PD: Alcohol-related skeletal disorders. *Ann NY Acad Sci* 1975;252:287–291.
25. Williams K: Introduction. Part VI. Infectious disease, in Seixas FA, Williams K, Eggleton S (eds): *Medical Consequences of Alcoholism*. New York, New York Academy of Sciences, 1975.
26. Heinemann HO: Alcohol and the lung: A brief review. *Am J Med* 1977;63:81–85.
27. Woeber K: The skin in diagnosis of alcoholism, in Seixas FA, Williams K, Eggleton S (eds): *Medical Consequences of Alcoholism*. New York, New York Academy of Sciences, 1975.
28. Hines JD: Effects of alcohol on inborn errors of metabolism: Porphyria cutanea tarda and hemochromatosis. *Semin Hematol* 1980;17:113–118.

17
Metabolic and Renal Effects of Alcohol

JENNIFER DALEY and JOHN T. HARRINGTON

Alcohol has a wide variety of renal and metabolic effects. Hepatic encephalopathy, peripheral neuropathy, and hyperglycemia secondary to pancreatic destruction can be considered metabolic in nature. However, in this chapter we narrow the definition and focus on four major acid–base and electrolyte disturbances due to alcohol—alcoholic ketoacidosis, hypomagnesemia, hypocalcemia, and hypophosphatemia—and on the hepatorenal syndrome, one of the major causes of renal failure in the severely ill, alcoholic patient with hepatic insufficiency.

Metabolic Disturbances

Alcoholic Ketoacidosis

The accumulation of ketoacids (beta-hydroxybutyrate and acetoacetate)[1-3] in body fluids is evidenced in three conditions: starvation, diabetic ketoacidosis, and alcoholic ketoacidosis.[4] Beta-hydroxybutyrate (BOHB) and acetoacetate (AcAc), the major ketone products, are produced by the liver almost exclusively and in equal amounts. Normally, blood levels of BOHB and AcAc are low (less than 0.1 mM/L). Starvation is the most common cause of ketosis worldwide, but the magnitude of ketosis from starvation is generally mild. Total fasting for at least one to two weeks is required to raise blood levels of BOBH and AcAc to more than 7.0 mM/L and more than 1.5 mM/L, respectively. Blood ketone levels rise as a result of increased hepatic production, decreased peripheral use, and enhanced renal conservation of ketoacids. During a one to two week period of fasting, renal ammoniagenesis increases sufficiently to offset the increase in endogenous acid production, and the plasma bicarbonate concentration stabilizes at slightly to moderately reduced levels. Plasma bicarbonate rarely falls below 17 mM/L as a result of pure starvation ketosis. Since poor dietary intake frequently accompanies acute or chronic alcoholism, starvation can contribute to the ketosis seen in the alcoholic patient.

It is well known that alcoholism causes ketosis,[4] but data are not available on the percentage of alcoholic patients admitted to inpatient units with ketosis. Frank metabolic ketoacidosis is unusual, for reasons that are not clear.[4]

Alcoholic ketoacidosis is seen in heavy drinkers who have been vomiting and have eaten little or no food for several days. The liver metabolizes alcohol into acetaldehyde and acetate. The acetate then stimulates hepatic production of ketoacids and, in particular, the production of BOHB. Because of alteration in the redox potential within cells, the BOHB:AcAc ratio is shifted in favor of BOHB in alcoholic ketoacidosis, similar to combined lactic and diabetic ketoacidosis (typically 3:1 to 4:1 in diabetic ketoacidosis). The bedside nitroprusside test (a drop of serial dilutions of serum or plasma placed on separate nitroprusside tablets, Acetest) measures AcAc and not BOHB. As a result, the bedside nitroprusside test in alcoholics with ketosis may be negative or mildly positive.[4]

Since serum BOHB and AcAc levels are not easily available clinically, the diagnosis of alcoholic ketoacidosis should be suspected in any alcoholic patient when the plasma bicarbonate level is low, the anion gap—defined as (Na) − ($Cl+HCO_3$)—is increased, the blood lactate level is not markedly elevated, and the nitroprusside test is weakly positive or negative. The blood sugar in these patients is usually less than 200 mg/dL.

The key therapeutic agents in the treatment of either alcoholic ketosis or frank ketoacidosis are glucose and sufficient sodium chloride and water to replace any volume and water deficits. Insulin therapy is not required in the majority of patients.[4] If we assume the patient has an intact endocrine pancreas, insulin levels will rise with glucose infusion. Ketoacid production will be cut off immediately, and blood ketone levels will fall to zero within hours.

Just as in the patient with diabetic ketoacidosis, plasma bicarbonate rises as a consequence of the metabolism of the ketoacids. Although ketoacidosis with low serum bicarbonate levels is the major metabolic, acid–base disorder in acute alcoholism, our experience indicates that respiratory alkalosis with secondary low serum bicarbonate is more common in patients with chronic alcoholism and cirrhosis. A blood pH determination is required to distinguish between these two acid–base disorders.

Alcoholics are prone to mixed acid–base disorders and can suffer from lactic acidosis due to septic shock (or alcohol itself), alcoholic ketoacidosis, respiratory alkalosis, and metabolic alkalosis from vomiting.[5] The clinical expression of such a complex derangement cannot be predicted and depends on the relative severity of the independent acid–base disorders (Table 17.1).

TABLE 17.1. Some common acid–base, electrolyte, and fluid disturbances in alcoholic patients.

Alcoholic ketoacidosis	Metabolic alkalosis secondary to vomiting and/or diuretics
Hypomagnesemia	Respiratory alkalosis
Hypocalcemia	Mixed acid–base disorders
Hypophosphatemia	Hypokalemia
Hyponatremia	Hypoglycemia
Hypernatremia	Hyperglycemia

Hypomagnesemia

Frequently, hypomagnesemia (serum level less than 1.4 mEq/L)[6-8] accompanies acute and chronic alcoholism, and at one time, it was thought to be responsible for many of the symptoms of delirium tremens. Magnesium, the second most common cation within cells, has a variety of action intracellularly. Thus, it is not surprising that moderate to severe hypomagnesemia results in a wide spectrum of clinical manifestations, including neuromuscular irritability, fatigue, and muscle weakness.[9] Serum magnesium concentration is usually maintained between 1.4 and 2.1 mEq/L (0.7 to 1.0 mM). Normal dietary intake of magnesium is approximately 300 mg/day (equal to 25 mEq), of which one third is absorbed from the gastrointestinal tract. The kidneys filter more than 3500 mg of magnesium each day, and maintenance of a steady state of magnesium balance demands that all the filtered magnesium be reabsorbed by the renal tubules. About 3% of the filtered load is excreted in the steady state (100 to 150 mg/day, 8 to 15 mEq), an amount equal to that absorbed from the gut each day.

Total body magnesium depletion (serum magnesium level of less than 1.0 mEq/L) can result from gastrointestinal malabsorption, decreased dietary intake, or renal tubular magnesium wasting. Decreased dietary intake of magnesium, when compounded by malabsorption, produces the largest contribution to total body magnesium depletion in alcoholics, especially those with poor protein–calorie intake. Alcohol has also been shown to increase renal magnesium excretion. In addition, the most widely used diuretic in current use, furosemide, depresses magnesium reabsorption by the nephron. Refeeding the alcoholic patient who is already protein–calorie deprived can cause a shift of magnesium into cells. Generally, serum magnesium levels are not available in standard chemistry screening panels, and hypomagnesemia may go undetected in the acutely ill alcoholic unless ordered specifically.

The interrelationships among magnesium, calcium, potassium, and phosphate are complex, but three interactions are important to recall when managing an alcoholic patient.[9] First, hypomagnesemia itself can cause renal potassium wasting. In the alcoholic patient with metabolic alkalosis, a more severe degree of potassium depletion may be seen because of the concomitant hypomagnesemia. Second, alcoholism can cause phosphate depletion, which results in renal tubular magnesium wasting, compounding the degree of magnesium depletion. Third, chronic hypomagnesemia suppresses parathyroid hormone (PTH) secretion, resulting in a decline in serum calcium. In a patient with a serum magnesium level less than 1 mEq/L, renal magnesium wasting can be documented by finding more than 5 mEq of magnesium in a 24-hour urine collection.

Treatment of hypomagnesemia requires either intravenous or oral repletion. In a patient with severe hypomagnesemia (less than 0.75 to 1 mEq/L) or with clinical symptoms (a positive Chvostek's sign or asterixis), 8 mEq of magnesium sulfate should be given intravenously (available as a 50% solution in a 2 ml ampule) every one to four hours until the serum magnesium level rises to 1 mEq/L. Orally, magnesium can be given as the glucoheptonate salt; 15 mL three times a day will supply 225 mg of elemental magnesium each day. Again, the dose should be adjusted according to the serum magnesium level.

Hypocalcemia

Hypocalcemia[10,11] of alcoholism results from at least two synergistic factors. First, chronic magnesium depletion suppresses PTH secretion, and the resultant hypoparathyroidism produces a fall in serum calcium levels. In alcoholic patients with hypocalcemia attributed to chronic magnesium deficiency, PTH levels should document this effect, since acute magnesium depletion stimulates PTH secretion. Second, chronic liver disease can impair the 25-hydroxylation of calciferol. In the alcoholic patient with poor dietary intake, decrease in vitamin D contributes to hypocalcemia by causing reduction in the amount of calcium absorbed from the gastrointestinal tract. Treatment of the alcoholic patient with symptomatic, significant hypocalcemia (less than 7 mg/dL) requires slow (not more than 10 ml/minute) intravenous administration of 10 mL of 10% calcium gluconate solution until symptoms clear or until the serum calcium rises above 7.5 mg/dL. Intravenous calcium chloride should not be used, since extravasation can cause local tissue necrosis. In mild hypocalcemia, correction of hypomagnesemia usually returns calcium levels to the normal range. In chronic cases, supplemental oral calcium can be given either as calcium carbonate, calcium gluconate, or calcium chloride until the serum calcium returns to normal.

Hypophosphatemia

The pathogenesis of hypophosphatemia[12,13] associated with alcoholism is as complex as that of hypomagnesemia and hypocalcemia. Hypophosphatemia due to an isolated dietary deficiency does not occur. Renal conservation of phosphate is stimulated when human volunteers are given oral phosphate binders and a low phosphorus intake. In those patients, urinary phosphate excretion falls to zero, and phosphate balance is virtually maintained.[14] Phosphate depletion in patients with alcoholism occurs for several reasons: gastrointestinal malabsorption of phosphate due to concomitant ketoacidosis, an increase in PTH secretion related to acute magnesium depletion in some patients, and, most importantly, a shift of phosphate into cells when glucose is administered.[14]

Mild to moderate hypophosphatemia (1 to 2 mg/dL) occurs in up to 50% of hospitalized patients and is not associated with either phosphate depletion or symptoms. However, severe hypophosphatemia (less than 1 mg/dL) is almost always associated with total body phosphate depletion.[1] Severe neuromuscular symptoms are present frequently, and ptosis, dysarthria, difficulty in swallowing, paresthesias, seizures, and respiratory failure have been noted. In addition, proximal muscle myopathy with rhabdomyolysis, depressed left ventricular function, and frank hemolysis have been described. The phosphate depletion syndrome can mimic delirium tremens, but hallucinations are absent in pure phosphate depletion. Recognizing that phosphate levels reach their nadir on the second to fourth hospital day, the physician should measure the plasma phosphate in every alcoholic patient admitted to the hospital. It is reasonable to add 20 to 40 mmol of potassium phosphate to each liter of fluid for patients with alcoholic ketoacidosis and other alcoholics receiving intravenous glucose solutions even before obtaining the results of the serum phosphate level. Until oral feedings are resumed, 100 to 120 mmol should be given daily. In the alcoholic receiving total parenteral nutrition, hypophosphatemia should be anticipated and potassium phosphate should be given prophylactically. Obviously, calcium salts and phosphate should not be administered through the same intravenous line, since precipitation of calcium phosphate will result.

Deficits in salt and water must be corrected in addition to restoring normal acid–base balance by administering glucose and restoring total body losses of magnesium, calcium, and phosphate. Patients with alcoholism are frequently volume depleted and may require 4 to 6 L of saline in the first 24 hours. Acute alcohol ingestion inhibits the secretion of ADH and leads to renal water loss. Unless this is replaced, hypernatremia can result.

Renal Effects of Alcohol: The Hepatorenal Syndrome

Patients with advanced cirrhosis and hepatic insufficiency may suffer from a peculiar functional type of renal failure, the hepatorenal syndrome.[15-17] The functional nature of the syndrome is best demonstrated by two dramatic clinical observations. When the kidneys of a patient dying of hepatorenal syndrome are transplanted into a host with normal hepatic function, they work normally, and when patients with hepatorenal syndrome undergo liver transplantation, the kidneys regain their normal function. It seems likely that this functional renal insufficiency results from intense renal vasoconstriction. Efforts to reverse the vasoconstriction with vasodilators have failed.

The hepatorenal syndrome occurs during the final stages of progressive hepatic insufficiency and is a grave prognostic sign. The patient is deeply jaundiced, with ascites, spider angioma, and signs of hepatic encephalopathy. A small gastrointestinal bleed, sepsis, or injudicious use of potent loop diuretics to treat fluid retention may precipitate renal failure. Serum creatinine and blood urea nitrogen rise slowly. Hyperkalemia is not a problem because of the severe secondary hyperaldosteronism present in end-stage hepatic failure. The urine sodium concentration is low (less than 5 mEq/L), and the urine specific gravity is greater than 1.020, reflecting intense renal ischemia. A thorough search for reversible causes of renal failure should be made (eg, intravascular salt and water depletion, urinary tract obstruction or infection, congestive heart failure, malignant hypertension, hypercalcemia, and acute tubular necrosis), and the medication record should be carefully reviewed for potential nephrotoxins.

Alcoholic patients with hepatic insufficiency and hepatorenal syndrome usually die from other complications of liver disease rather than of renal failure. Hemodialysis is indicated only if there is a reasonable hope for survival.

Given the bleak prognosis, prevention of the hepatorenal syndrome by careful attention to drug selection and maintenance of an adequate intravascular volume provide the only sound approach to the management of the patient with severe hepatic insufficiency.

Acknowledgment. Research for this chapter was supported in part by a grant from the Robert Wood Johnson Foundation.

References

1. Halperin ML, Hammeke M, Josse RG, Jungas RL: Metabolic acidoses in the alcoholic: A pathophysiologic approach. *Metabolism* 1983;32:308–315.
2. Kreisberg RA, Owen WC, Siegal AM: Ethanol-induced hyperlactic acidemia: Inhibition of lactate utilization. *J Clin Invest* 1971;50:166–174.
3. DeMarchi S, Cecchin E: Alcoholic ketoacidosis. *Br Med J* 1986;292:960.
4. Cahill GF Jr: Nephrology Forum. Ketosis. *Kidney Int* 1982;20:416–425.
5. Harrington JT, Cohen JJ, Kassirer JP: Mixed acid–base disturbances, in Cohen JJ, Kassirer JP (eds): *Acid–Base*. Boston, Little, Brown, and Company, 1982.
6. Whang R: Magnesium deficiency: Causes and clinical implications. *Drugs* 1984;28 (suppl 1):143–150.
7. Ryzen E, Wagers PW, Singer FR, Fude RK: Magnesium deficiency in a medical ICU population. *Crit Care Med* 1985;13:19–21.
8. Berkelhammer C, Bear RA: A clinical approach to common electrolyte problems. 4. Hypomagnesemia. *Can Med Assoc J* 1985;132:360–368.
9. Dirks JH: Nephrology Forum. The kidney and magnesium regulation. *Kidney Int* 1983;23:771–777.
10. Stevenson JC: Fluid and electrolyte disorders. Calcium. *Br J Hosp Med* 1984;32:71–72, 75–76.
11. Favus MJ: Factors that influence absorption and secretion of calcium in the small intestine and colon. *Am J Physiol* 1985;248:G147–G157.
12. Lotz M, Zisman E, Bartter FC: Evidence of a phosphorus depletion syndrome in man. *N Engl J Med* 1968;278:409–415.
13. Newman JH, Neff TA, Ziporin PH: Acute respiratory failure associated with hypophosphatemia. *N Engl J Med* 1977;296:1101–1103.
14. Ritz E: Nephrology Forum. Acute hypophosphatemia. *Kidney Int* 1981;22:89–94.
15. Zipsser R, Hoefs P, Speckart P, et al: Evidence for a critical role of prostaglandins in renin release, vascular reactivity and renal function in liver disease. *J Clin Endocrinol Metab* 1979;48:895.
16. Levenson DJ, Skorecki KL, Narins RG: Acute renal failure associated with hepatobiliary disease, in Brenner BM, Lazarus JM (eds): *Acute Renal Failure*. Philadelphia, WB Saunders, 1983.
17. Popper S: Hepatorenal syndrome, in Epstein M (ed): *The Kidney in Liver Disease*. New York, Elsevier, 1983.

18
Alcoholism and Cancer

JOAN SAVITSKY

In addition to the better-known miseries associated with alcoholism, there is also an increased incidence of certain types of cancer among alcoholics. The best-established association is with head and neck cancers, although cancer at a number of other sites, particularly primary hepatocellular carcinoma, has been attributed to alcoholism. It is unclear whether alcoholics have an overall increased risk of dying from cancer. Breeden[1] estimates that 10% to 20% increased cancer mortality can be directly attributable to alcohol. However, data from Schmidt and Popham[2] do not show an overall increase in cancer mortality. Rothman estimates that about 3% of all cancers in the United States in 1974 could be attributed to alcohol.[3] Understanding both the epidemiology and the mechanisms relating cancer and alcohol is confounded by the use of cigarettes (often accompanying heavy alcohol use) and the omnipresent difficulty of obtaining an accurate history of alcohol use.

Head and Neck Cancers

Cancers originating in the oral cavity are strongly associated with both drinking and smoking. This makes sense intuitively, since the structures of the oral cavity are in close proximity to the offending substances. However, the actual mechanism for this association is speculative. Alcohol, by itself, is associated with an increased risk of oral cancer. Rothman's data[3] showed that the relative risk for carcinoma of the mouth and pharynx went from 1.0 for the nonsmoking nondrinker to 2.3 for the nonsmoking drinker who consumed over 1.5 ounces of alcohol (approximately three to four drinks) per day. The combination of smoking and drinking may be synergistic in its carcinogenic potential. According to Rothman, the heavy drinker who smokes over two packs per day has a relative risk of 15.5 for oral cancer. He estimates that alcohol and tobacco together are responsible for 75% of oral cancers in American males.[3]

Both oral and esophageal cancers seem related more to drinking than to the use of tobacco.[4,5] Laryngeal cancer, on the other hand, is more strongly associated with cigarettes.[5,6] In fact, the nonsmoking heavy drinker has no increase in risk of laryngeal malignancy. For the moderate or heavy smoker, however, increasing use of alcohol does multiply the risk of this cancer.[6]

Esophageal cancer is closely connected with heavy drinking but has been related to other factors, including the type of alcoholic beverage consumed, cigarette smoking, diet, and a history of lye ingestion. Heavy drinkers have a 20-fold increased incidence over nondrinkers.[3] Tuyns has demonstrated an epidemiologic association between esophageal cancer and rates of alcoholism in certain regions of France.[7,8] Both Tuyns and Rothman observed that the exceptionally high incidence of esophageal cancer in certain areas of the world is suggestive of an additional cause (perhaps a contaminant in the local beverage) beyond the use of alcohol alone.[3,8]

As with other cancers, the role of cigarettes is hard to separate from that of alcohol. As an independent factor, the effect of smoking has been estimated to vary from strong to insignificant by different authors.[1,6,9,10] Schmidt and deLint cite the interesting observation (made in 1910 when the use of cigarettes was relatively rare) that "absinthism" was noted in 80% of patients with cancer of the esophagus and cardia.[11]

Hepatocellular Carcinoma

Hepatocellular carcinoma (HCC) or hepatoma, relatively uncommon in the United States, is far more common in other parts of the world and is usually associated with chronic hepatitis B viral (HBV) infection. In the United States, hepatoma occurs most often in the setting of alcoholic cirrhosis. Among patients with hepatoma, the incidence of underlying cirrhosis from any cause is estimated at 16% to 80%.[12] The true incidence is probably closer to the higher number. Omata et al found that when hepatoma occurs in alcoholic liver disease there is a background of advanced cirrhosis.[13]

Rothman points out that, although hepatoma is strongly associated with alcoholic cirrhosis, cohort studies of mortality among alcoholics do not reflect this.[3] The reason is unclear, especially since an autopsy study by Lee showed that in 84 alcoholics with cirrhosis, 25 (30%) had hepatoma.[14] This study also found an increased incidence of hepatoma among those alcoholics who had curtailed their drinking some time before death. Lee speculates that this may be due to either (1) increased survival of the abstinent alcoholic, permitting development of supervening hepatoma, or (2) an inhibitory effect on hepatoma of continued heavy drinking.

A number of investigators have explored the role of chronic HBV infection in this process. Bréchot et al in France found that in their study all 20 alcoholics with hepatocellular carcinoma had evidence of HBV DNA integrated into the genome of neoplastic liver cells, compared to a 16% incidence in alcoholics without hepatocellular carcinoma.[15] They concluded that alcohol may act as a cocarcinogen with chronic HBV infection. In addition, Bréchot and a number of others have noted an increased incidence of positive HBV serologies in alcoholic subjects.[15-17] Some have suggested that alcoholics be immunized against type B hepatitis before exposure in order to minimize the risk of eventual hepatoma.[15,16] Ohnishi et al observed that even modest use of alcohol may accelerate the development of hepatoma in carriers of Hb_sAg. This led them to suggest that these people not use any alcohol.[18]

Inconclusive Data

The increased mortality from lung cancer in alcoholics is probably entirely due to the associated use of cigarettes.[2] The pancreas would seem intuitively to be a site for malignant transformation in the chronic alcoholic, but data on this subject are conflicting.[19-21] Similarly unclear at present is an association between alcoholism and carcinoma of the colon,[2,5,11] rectum,[22,23] prostate,[5,9,11] stomach,[5,11,24] and thyroid[5] and malignant melanoma.[5] Two recent studies suggest that moderate alcohol intake (one or more drinks daily) is associated with an increased risk of breast cancer in women.[25,26]

Mechanisms

Many different mechanisms have been proposed to explain the association between alcohol and malignancy. Some are speculative; others have experimental or epidemiologic backing. The same mechanism probably does not account for all cancers, and a number of different ones acting in concert may be responsible. The most obvious explanation is that, like tobacco, alcohol itself is a carcinogen. There is little evidence to support this contention, although alcohol does injure tissue, and the response of cellular proliferation may predispose to neoplastic change, as is hypothesized in the case of hepatoma.

If not itself a carcinogen, alcohol may function as a cocarcinogen by enhancing the effect of other agents. It may act as either a solvent or a local irritant, augmenting entry of the actual carcinogen into the underlying tissue. However, this would explain cancers only in sites that come into direct contact with alcohol, such as the oropharynx. Alcohol may have systemic activity as a cocarcinogen via its metabolic effect of inducing microsomal enzyme systems in the liver and other tissues.[27] This, in turn, enhances the conversion of certain procarcinogens to carcinogens. Alternatively, the cirrhotic liver, which is compromised in its housecleaning function, may be less able to detoxify circulating carcinogens.

It is possible that alcohol has no role in tumor induction but promotes the growth of an established tumor. It may not be alcohol itself but some contaminant in alcoholic beverages that is related to the development of cancer. This would be consistent with some (admittedly conflicting) epidemiologic data that suggest that certain cancers are more strongly associated with one particular type of beverage alcohol.

Since alcoholism exists in a complex web of associated problems and conditions, the increased rate of malignancy could be attributable to any of these other problems. The most obvious is the heavy use of cigarettes, although most epidemiologic studies have attempted to control for smoking. Another potential mechanism is the malnutrition that frequently accompanies alcoholism. There is experimental evidence that malnourished mice are more susceptible to the development of tumors,[6] and there is the clinical example of the Plummer-Vinson syndrome in which iron-deficient women are prone to pharyngeal carcinoma.

Alcoholics frequently have poor dentition, which changes the oral flora and, in turn, may increase local carcinogens. Their immune system is often compromised, potentially increasing the risk for neoplasia as in other immunocompromised populations. Both these mechanisms are speculative and difficult to establish epidemiologically in large studies, but they are intuitively appealing and illustrate the potential complexity of the interactions.

Treatment

Clinical problems encountered when caring for the cancer patient with coexisting alcoholism include postoperative delirium tremens, noncompliance, and fewer psychosocial resources for coping and support. In addition, treating the alcoholic patient often involves the use of antineoplastic drugs and radiotherapy, less well tolerated by the already compromised alcoholic. Breeden notes that pancytopenia (frequently dose-limiting in the use of these agents) may be encountered earlier in alcoholic patients due to underlying bone marrow suppression, folate and other nutritional deficiencies, and hypersplenism.[1] He cautions that patients taking procarbazine and alcohol together may have a disulfiram-like reaction. Alcohol may enhance the toxicities of some antineoplastic drugs and radiation. Laboratory evidence shows that cancer cells are sensitized to bleomycin cytotoxicity when exposed to alcohol just before or following treatment. The explanation is speculative: bleomycin may damage the cellular DNA, and repair mechanisms may be inhibited by alcohol. Alternatively, alcohol may potentiate bleomycin activity in the cells.[28]

Discussion

The alcoholic patient is definitely at risk for head and neck cancers, probably at risk for primary hepatocellular carcinoma, and possibly at risk for other cancers. Further epidemiologic studies are needed to clarify the full spectrum of alcohol-associated malignancies. Once the alcoholic has developed a malignancy, more than the usual management problems are encountered because of preexisting physical and psychosocial difficulties.

References

1. Breeden JH: Alcohol, alcoholism, and cancer. *Med Clin North Am* 1984;68:163–177.
2. Schmidt W, Popham RE: The role of drinking and smoking in mortality from cancer and other causes in male alcoholics. *Cancer* 1981;47:1031–1041.
3. Rothman KJ: The proportion of cancer attributable to alcohol consumption. *Prev Med* 1980;9:174–179.
4. Mashberg A, Garfinkle L, Harris S: Alcohol as a primary risk factor in oral squamous carcinoma. *CA* 1981;31:146–155.
5. Williams RR, Horm JW: Association of cancer sites with tobacco and alcohol consumption and socioeconomic status of patients: Interview study from the Third National Cancer Survey. *J Natl Cancer Inst* 1977;58:525–547.
6. McCoy GD, Wynder EL: Etiological and preventive implications in alcohol carcinogenesis. *Cancer Res* 1979;39:2844–2850.
7. Tuyns AJ: Cancer of the oesophagus: Further evidence of the relation to drinking habits in France. *Int J Cancer* 1970;5:152–156.
8. Tuyns AJ, Massé LMF: Mortality from cancer of the oesophagus in Brittany. *Int J Epidemiol* 1973;2:241–245.
9. National Institute for Alcoholism and Alcohol Abuse (NIAAA): Alcohol and cancer, in *Alcohol and Health. 2nd Special Report to Congress*. DHEW, 1974:69–90.
10. Wynder EL, Bross IJ: A study of etiological factors in cancer of the esophagus. *Cancer* 1961;14:389–413.
11. Schmidt W, deLint J: Causes of death of alcoholics. *Q J Stud Alcohol* 1972;33: 171–185.
12. Chan CH: Primary carcinoma of the liver. *Med Clin North Am* 1975;59:989–994.
13. Omata M, Ashcavai M, Liew C, Peters RL: Hepatocellular carcinoma in the USA, etiologic considerations. *Gastroenterology* 1979;76:279–287.
14. Lee FI: Cirrhosis and hepatoma in alcoholics. *Gut* 1966;7:77–85.
15. Bréchot C, et al: Evidence that hepatitis B virus has a role in liver-cell carcinoma in alcoholic liver disease. *N Engl J Med* 1982;306:1384–1387.
16. Goudeau A, et al: Hepatitis B infection in alcoholic liver disease and primary hepatocellular carcinoma in France. *Prog Med Virol* 1981;27:26–34.
17. Mills PR, et al: Evidence for previous hepatitis B virus infection in alcoholic cirrhosis. *Br Med J* 1981;282:437–438.
18. Ohnishi K, et al: The effect of chronic habitual alcohol intake on the development of liver cirrhosis and hepatocellular carcinoma: Relation to hepatitis B surface antigen carriage. *Cancer* 1982;49:672–677.
19. Berg JW, Connelly RR: Updating the epidemiologic data on pancreatic cancer. *Semin Oncol* 1979;6:275–284.
20. Burch GE, Ansari A: Chronic alcoholism and carcinoma of the pancreas. *Arch Intern Med* 1968;122:273–275.
21. Monson RR, Lyon JL: Proportional mortality among alcoholics. *Cancer* 1975;36: 1077–1079.
22. Breslow NE, Enstrom JE: Geographic correlates between cancer mortality rates and alcohol-tobacco consumption in the United States. *J Natl Cancer Inst* 1974;53: 631–639.
23. Tuyns AJ: Epidemiology of alcohol and cancer. *Cancer Res* 1979;39:2840–2843.

24. Klatsky AL, Friedman GD, Siegelaub AB: Alcohol and mortality, a ten-year Kaiser-Permanente experience. *Ann Intern Med* 1981;95:139–145.
25. Schatzkin A, Jones DY, Hoover RN, et al: Alcohol consumption and breast cancer in the epidemiologic follow-up study of the First National Health and Nutrition Examination Survey. *N Engl J Med* 1987;316:1169–1173.
26. Willett WC, Stampfer MJ, Colditz GA, et al: Moderate alcohol consumption and the risk of breast cancer. *N Engl J Med* 1987;316:1174–1179.
27. MacSween RNM: Alcohol and cancer. *Br Med Bull* 1982;38:31–33.
28. Mizuno S: Ethanol-induced cell sensitization to bleomycin toxicity and the inhibition of recovery from potentially lethal damage. *Cancer Res* 1981;41:4111–4114.

Part VI Alcohol and Special Populations

In this section, we focus on the special difficulties alcohol poses for the family, the elderly, women, adolescent drinkers, and physicians and address also the issues particular to those people who abuse multiple substances. We believe that these six special populations hold particular relevance for the primary physician.

In discussing the family and alcoholism, the Griners focus on several phenomena often ignored by the practitioner. They point out that the prevalence of codependency may be as high as 25% in this country, how denial exists within the entire family, and the importance of viewing alcoholism as a family illness. They give striking examples of how the physician may educate and encourage the family to participate in a structured intervention, an important step toward successful recovery. One of the sad ironies is that, as the alcoholic patient improves, the family becomes increasingly at risk.

Hesse and Savitsky discuss the obstacles involved in screening the elderly for alcoholism. They focus on the constellation of problems that may lead to the geriatric squalor syndrome and stress how difficult it is to differentiate cognitive degeneration related to a myriad of causes from loss of function related primarily to alcohol abuse. They point to the differences in natural history and response to therapy of those who begin to drink heavily late in life, in contrast to those who start early.

The chapter by Halliday and Bush notes that women generally start to drink heavily later than their male counterparts but that problems with alcohol among employed women appear to be on the increase. They stress the pitfalls in establishing a diagnosis in women and point to special approaches needed when treating women.

Bean-Bayog highlights the special problems that the adolescent poses for the practitioner. Although the common physiologic manifestations of alcoholism may be absent, the relation of alcohol to death by accident in the young is an important reason for aggressive intervention by the doctor and family. This chapter stresses the tendency toward multiple drug abuse, since adolescents rarely drink heavily without using other drugs. She discusses how attitudes toward alcoholism and illness may be very different in the adolescent. Unless this is understood, difficulties in diagnosis and treatment may result.

Although recent data suggest that physicians are at no higher risk of alcohol abuse than are other adults or professionals, they do pose a special problem to colleagues and patients. Spickard reports that physicians frequently combine alcohol abuse with abuse of meperidine and other drugs. He shows how colleagues of the physician may collude, albeit unconsciously, in protecting the ill individual from intervention. Spickard gives concrete examples of how to bring the physician into therapy.

In addressing the issue of patients suffering from mixed-substance abuse, Bayog reminds us that alcoholism rarely occurs without the use of other drugs and, conversely, that the use of marijuana, cocaine, heroin, or other drugs is frequently accompanied by alcohol abuse. He stresses the nature of the physician-patient relationship and describes different forms of therapy available to patients who abuse multiple substances.

19
Alcoholism and the Family

MIRIAM E. GRINER and PAUL F. GRINER

Many physicians perceive the typical alcoholic as one who exists largely in isolation, having lost contact with family and friends, and essentially without any social support system. In reality, the majority of alcoholics exist within intact family structures. The effects of the alcoholic on the family are profound, resulting in significant functional impairment of these family members, often termed "codependents." As Wegscheider has stated, "few alcoholics play out their drama alone. Like the embattled protagonist of a Shakespearean tragedy, blind and unknowing, they take a whole cast of supporting characters down with them."[1]

If one accepts an estimate of 10% for the prevalence of alcoholism in adults, the prevalence of codependency is probably no less than 25%. This is a staggering figure, particularly when one recognizes that codependents suffer varying levels of dysfunction often unrecognized and untreated.

Although this chapter addresses the effect of the alcoholic on the codependent, the impact of the codependent's behavior on the alcoholic is of equal importance. The family that does not understand alcoholism will enable the disease to continue. Families of alcoholics must recognize the illness early in its course, know that effective treatment is available, and participate in intervention and treatment. Treatment before the family unit has been destroyed is associated with improved long-term outcomes for alcoholics.[2] It is only in recent years, however, that the importance of the family in the treatment of the alcoholic has been recognized. The *Second Special Report to the US Congress on Alcohol and Health* referred to family therapy of alcoholism as "the most notable current advance" in the treatment and rehabilitation of the alcoholic.[3]

Impact of the Alcoholic on the Family

Families tend to react in patterned and predictable ways when one member becomes alcoholic. Over a number of years, the family moves from the supportive relationships that characterize the healthy family toward an increasingly dysfunctional state. The observations of Jackson,[4] Wegscheider,[1] and Black[5] reinforce the findings that people undergoing the same type of stress under similar circumstances often show similar types of abnormal and adaptive behavior patterns. In alcoholic families, certain patterns, such as denial, secretiveness, lack of honesty, and suppression of feelings, are observed with remarkable consistency.

Denial among codependents can be a powerful but maladaptive defense and may for many years prevent the spouse of an alcoholic from recognizing the root cause of a deteriorating marital relationship. This mechanism is more pronounced among the husbands of alcoholic women than vice versa.[6] Denial may be so pervasive that when a physician attempts to confirm a history of excessive alcoholic intake from the spouse of a patient exhibiting an obvious medical complication of alcoholism, the spouse may unconsciously mislead the physician into seeking another cause for the medical problem. The importance of recognizing denial is underscored by the observation that the spouse of the alcoholic may become convinced that he or she is the cause of a deteriorating marriage. Should the spouse seek out the physician for counseling, the history will likely be highly distorted.

Once family members recognize that a spouse, parent, or child has alcoholism, they develop coping strategies designed to ensure the integrity of the family unit. They do not discuss the problem among themselves or with outsiders. Painful observations of alcoholic behavior are not shared; rather, family members hide the problem and their reactions from each other. A wife, physically abused by her alcoholic husband, will tell her children that she fell. She may suppress her own feelings in order to remain in an untenable situation.

The isolation of individual family members is compounded by the social isolation of the entire family. Children stop inviting friends over because of the unpredictability of an alcoholic parent's behavior. A spouse will refuse social invitations or make excuses for the alcoholic's absence from work. These behavior patterns of codependents – denial, secretiveness, lack of honesty, and suppression of feelings – are remarkably similar and parallel to those of the alcoholic. They serve to reinforce the fact that codependency is an illness requiring recognition and treatment as a primary entity.

As the family becomes increasingly preoccupied with the family member's drinking, there are attempts to reorganize, and various adaptive roles are developed. These roles have been classified by Wegscheider into the following basic patterns: the enabler, the hero, the scapegoat, the lost child, and the mascot.[1] For the physician, the importance of this classification lies not only in the insight it provides about the dynamics of the alcoholic family but also in the signs and symptoms of physical, mental, and behavioral problems that may ultimately be associated with each. The enabler, most often the spouse, takes over control of the family and assumes responsibilities previously held by the alcoholic. This family member is often perceived as stoic and strong-willed. He or she may be reluctant to seek care from a physician for illness until it has progressed to the point of incapacity. The hero, often the oldest child, is a high achiever who may ultimately go to the physician with anxiety or depression. The scapegoat may fall into a pattern of delinquency and self-destructive behavior. This member of the family is at high risk of addiction. The lost child, who tries to escape from the problem, may become withdrawn or schizoid. The mascot is one who seeks attention, demonstrates immature behavior, and may be a poor learner in school.

Often the behavior of these children brings them to professional attention before alcoholism is diagnosed in a parent or other family member. The impact of an alcoholic parent on the children can be devastating. Although detailed discussion of the consequences is beyond the scope of this book, several points should be stressed relative to the children of an alcoholic parent. First, the extent to which a child is affected depends on which parent is alcoholic, how sick the alcoholic is, and the age of the child when the alcoholism has progressed to the point of family disruption. The younger the child when drinking begins, the more serious is its impact on the child's subsequent adult life.[6] In general, an alcoholic mother is more damaging to the child than an alcoholic father. Second, interviews with children of alcoholic families show that they share the feelings described by the spouse of the alcoholic: shame, fear, anger, resentment, confusion, and emotional isolation.[7] They lack trust and often have difficulty establishing relationships outside the family. Third, perhaps of greatest concern, is the high frequency with which children of alcoholics subsequently become addicted to alcohol or other drugs. For further discussion, the reader is referred to the excellent descriptions in articles by Estes and Heinemann[6] and Cork[7] and a pamphlet by the Johnson Institute.[8] Resources available to the children of an alcoholic parent are described later in this chapter.

Physicians who uncover an underlying problem of alcoholism by recognizing these behavior patterns among their patients are in a position to provide valuable assistance to the family and the problem drinker. Those who do not recognize these clues will unwittingly enable the primary problem and its impact on the family to continue.

Eventually the family's coping mechanisms fail, and efforts are made to escape the problem. Separation and divorce are the usual mechanisms. Women who do not have independent financial resources may find it more difficult to escape, particularly when they are responsible for raising children. Tragically, in some cases, suicide becomes the means of escape.

During this late stage when breakup of the family is imminent, it is common for the spouse to receive conflicting advice from other family members, friends, and social agencies. Some may counsel the spouse to leave; others, particularly those with a primary concern for the rehabilitation of the alcoholic, may counsel the spouse to remain. Should the spouse come to the physician for advice at this time, it is important that he maintain a neutral position and attempt to refer the spouse to a counselor, therapist, or agency with special expertise in the evaluation and treatment of families of alcoholics.

Impact of the Family on the Alcoholic

The extent to which the well-meaning, but uninformed, family's response to the alcoholic inhibits rather than facilitates recovery deserves special emphasis. Family members, for example, usually do not understand alcoholism as an addiction. Their approach to the alcoholic member is based most often on moral grounds—an approach as fruitless as it is uninformed. Neither reason nor threats are antidotes to the problem of drug dependence. Thus, kindness on the one hand or anger on the other are more likely to accelerate than reduce drinking by an alcoholic already suffering from low self-esteem. Similarly, the spouse who progressively assumes responsibilities previously held by the alcoholic or who protects the alcoholic by making excuses or by otherwise covering up for his behavior unwittingly enables the alcoholic to continue to drink. These well-intentioned approaches are ultimately destructive because they fail to address the need for alcoholics to face the consequences of their behavior as a prerequisite to treatment and eventual recovery. Protecting the alcoholic from the impact of his disease on others (most particularly the family) prolongs the disease and runs the risk of permitting both social and economic deterioration and medical complications to progress.[8]

In our experience, the concept that the alcoholic must face the consequences of his actions is one of the most difficult to accept, not only for families but for physicians as well. The distinction between an angry outburst and an honest, frank presentation by the spouse of the impact of the alcoholic's behavior is an important one. The former is counterproductive. The latter may begin to lead to acknowledgment of the problem, a necessary first step to recovery. Physicians who fail to recognize this distinction may enable the alcoholic to continue to drink if they counsel the spouse not to disturb the status quo when advice is sought about how to handle the problem. Similarly, the physician who treats the complications of alcoholism but fails to address the underlying problem is enabling the patient to continue a pattern of destructive drinking.

The Role of the Family in Intervention

Chapters 6 and 7 discussed various approaches to having the alcoholic accept the diagnosis. One of these is a structured intervention. The goal of an intervention is to show the alcoholic that he is unable to control his drinking. The process involves presenting to the alcoholic the negative effects of his drinking behavior on family members or close associates. This process rejects the principle that recovery from alcoholism cannot be expected until the alcoholic has hit bottom and realizes, spontaneously, that a problem exists that he must address. Intervention based on the assumption that the progression of physical and mental complications of alcoholism can be aborted provides the opportunity for a return to productive life through a process of confrontation and support. The confrontation is best organized by a professional counselor skilled in the conduct of interventions. To be successful, interventions must (1) actively involve those closest to the problem drinker, (2) present the alcoholic with a choice of either accepting that a drinking problem exists or being prepared to suffer a specific consequence, for example, loss of family or job, and (3) make available immediate treatment.

It is obvious that involvement of the family is crucial if an intervention is to succeed, whether it is conducted at the home or workplace. Family intervention provides the opportunity for the most important people in the alcoholic's life to demonstrate the impact of his actions on them, calling upon specific examples for reinforcement. One of the keys to the successful intervention is the presentation of alternatives to the impaired family member; that is, he must either recognize a drinking problem and undertake treatment for the problem or be prepared for the alternative. A common alternative is for the family to be prepared to leave if the alcoholic does not acknowledge that a drinking problem requiring treatment exists. The family must resolve to follow through with this alternative, as difficult as it may seem, because otherwise the intervention will lack the leverage needed for success. Although this approach may appear to be cruel and unfeeling, it must be compared with the probability of progressive deterioration of the alcoholic if drinking continues unabated.

There are obvious risks associated with intervention, but the unpublished experiences of many counselors skilled in the conduct of intervention suggest a surprisingly high success rate. Such interventions have become an integral component of employee-assistance programs in industries throughout the country. The physician who is involved in the early detection of alcoholism and its management needs to be aware of intervention as a therapeutic maneuver and know that community resources exist to help the family prepare for such an approach.

The Family in the Treatment of the Alcoholic

In an excellent article on family treatment approaches to alcoholism, Steinglass points out that involvement of the family in the treatment of the alcoholic has lagged behind the recognition of the magnitude of alcohol abuse and its impact on family members.[9] His article reviews the experimental and clinical literature on family treatment approaches over a 25-year period. It points out that treatment that involves the spouse of the alcoholic appears superior to either individual therapy or therapy limited to groups of alcoholics. Alcoholics in stable marital or work situations are known to have a more favorable response to treatment than those without these resources. The role of the intact family in facilitating the recovery of the alcoholic cannot be overemphasized.[10]

Involvement of the family in the treatment of the alcoholic is associated with improved sobriety, improved quality and functioning of the marriage, and increased well-being among the family members.[9] As Steinglass points out, caution must be used in interpreting the results of studies comparing various approaches to family therapy with those directed exclusively at the alcoholic, since most studies have significant methodologic flaws. On the other hand, it is difficult to argue with the point that alcoholism is indeed a family affair. Active involvement by the family of the alcoholic is intuitively sound.

Approaches to family therapy include individual treatment of the couple, group treatment with multiple couples, and treatment programs where spouses and children join the alcoholic member for up to a week at a treatment center, with follow-up group therapy for the couple after the alcoholic spouse returns home. A typical family week at a treatment center would include first an interview with each of the family members to assess their level of understanding of alcoholism. Didactic presentations concerning the pharmacology of alcohol and the pathophysiology and psychopathology of alcohol abuse follow. Interfamily group sessions are helpful for sharing experiences, for recognizing that the alcoholic's problem is truly a family problem, and for breaking down defenses that family members have developed to insulate themselves. This leads to increased awareness of the impact of the alcoholic's behavior on the family's ability to function effectively. Properly supervised confrontations between the alcoholic and involved family members are helpful in releasing long-standing anger and resentment. They help reestablish communication and lead both parties to better insights into each other's interests and needs. Commonly, weekly group sessions involving multiple couples are conducted for up to six months after the alcoholic has returned from the treatment center. The purpose of these aftercare programs is to help solidify the recovery of both partners that was initiated in the treatment center. The interested reader is referred to an excellent article by Usher et al describing the important phases in the course of family therapy of alcoholism.[11]

Treatment of the Codependent

Treatment of the family member of the alcoholic is important for numerous reasons. First, as indicated earlier, most family members do not recognize the extent to which their responses to the alcoholic have resulted in dysfunctional behavior (ie, isolation, enabling), depression, anxiety, or physical illness. Thus, treatment of the codependent is important in and of itself regardless of whether or not the alcoholic is in a recovery program.[10] Second, without better understanding of alcoholism and the impact of the alcoholic on the involved family member, it is common for spouses of alcoholics to remarry alcoholics or for sons or daughters of an alcoholic parent to marry an alcoholic.[8]

Third, education and treatment of the codependent help set the groundwork for the return of a normal family life during the recovery of the alcoholic. For example, Jackson has shown that for a couple facing a sober marriage after many years of drinking, expectations for the marriage may be unrealistic.[4] Her work recognizes that sustained recovery may require long-term commitment to the activities and principles of Alcoholics Anonymous. The recovered alcoholic may throw himself so heavily into AA that the codependent may sense competition from a new partner. The recovered alcoholic must be given responsibility for again assuming roles relinquished while drinking that were progressively assumed by the spouse or children. The spouse, in particular, may find it difficult to relinquish such roles. It is thus paradoxical that the integrity of the marriage may be at greatest risk during early recovery. These examples point out the changing dynamics of family life in recovery and reinforce the importance of attention to individual members' needs to grow and develop through education and treatment while the alcoholic is in recovery.

Finally, long-term health in children of an alcoholic parent is more likely if the whole family participates in treatment.[6] Those people involved in the social or medical evaluation and management of children should be well informed about problems encountered by the children of alcoholics and the availability of community resources to address these problems. Children who have been reared in a family where one or both parents are alcoholic may have never experienced a normal family life. They may require a lengthy period of treatment for their recovery.

Two useful treatment resources are family therapy programs offered by many alcohol treatment centers and the self-help groups, Al-Anon for adults and Alateen for children. Whereas family therapy programs may vary in approach and in coverage by health insurance policies, Al-Anon and Alateen meetings adhere to the principles and form of AA and are open to anyone whose life is affected by another person's drinking. These meetings recognize that the problems and needs of the codependent are similar to those of the alcoholic. Anecdotal experiences suggest that these self-help groups do indeed facilitate the physical and emotional well-being of the family member of the alcoholic, regardless of whether or not the alcoholic is continuing to drink. Continued attendance at Al-Anon meetings helps reinforce and sustain the recovery of the codependent.

Frequently, physicians care for codependent patients who continue to live with an actively drinking alcoholic. The physician's first task is to assess the codependent's degree of insight into the situation. Despite an assertion of "knowing all about alcoholism," codependents usually have distorted perceptions and basic misunderstandings about the nature of the disease. Although referral to a specific alcohol education group or to Al-Anon will address these issues, many codependent patients refuse such a referral, asserting that the problem is the alcoholic's and not theirs.

The physician can be helpful to these patients by using many of the strategies outlined in Chapter 6 for working with the denying patient. Some of the precepts of AA and Al-Anon can be incorporated into discussions in the office. Simply allowing the codependent to ventilate feelings about living with an alcoholic family member can counteract some of the sense of isolation. Because codependents often share the same feelings of powerlessness as the alcoholic, they may need help in understanding that they do in fact have choices about their relationship with the alcoholic. The primary care physician is in a position to remind the codependent gently that he must take responsibility for his own life, just as the alcoholic must take responsibility for his drinking. As in the care of the alcoholic, the course of the codependent family member will have periods of exacerbation when intervention may be more successful. Understanding the role that alcohol and the alcoholic play in the life of the codependent will be helpful in the assessment of other medical problems.

An informed and perceptive physician will (1) understand alcoholism as a family illness, (2) detect alcoholism through its impact on family members, (3) be aware of the unique stresses on the family at the time of intervention and early recovery, and (4) recognize the value of family therapy (including self-help groups) for the recovery of both alcoholics and their dependents.

Acknowledgment. We are grateful to Shirley Connell, CAC, for her insights and advice during the preparation of this manuscript.

References

1. Wegscheider S: *Another Chance.* Palo Alto, Science and Behavior Books, Inc, 1981.
2. Bromet E, Moos RH: Environmental resources and the posttreatment functioning of alcoholic patients. *J Health Soc Behav* 1977;18:326.
3. Keller M (ed): Trends in treatment of alcoholism, in *Second Special Report to the US Congress on Alcohol and Health.* DHEW, 1974:145–167.
4. Jackson JK: The adjustment of the family to the crisis of alcoholism. *J Q Stud Alcohol* 1954;15:562–586.
5. Black C: *It Will Never Happen to Me.* Denver, Medical Administration Company, 1982.
6. Estes N, Heinemann M (eds): *Alcoholism, Development, Consequences, and Interventions*, ed 2. St. Louis, CV Mosby Co, 1982.
7. Cork RM: *The Forgotten Children.* Don Mills, Ontario, Paper Jacks, 1969.
8. Johnson Institute Inc: *Chemical Dependency and Recovery Are a Family Affair.* Minneapolis, Johnson Institute Inc, 1979.
9. Steinglass P: Experimenting with family treatment approaches to alcoholism, 1950–1975: A review. *Fam Process* 1976;15:97–123.
10. Johnson VE: *I'll Quit Tomorrow: A Practical Guide to Alcoholism*, rev ed. San Francisco, Harper & Row, 1980.
11. Usher ML, Jay J, Glass DR: Family therapy as a treatment modality for alcoholism. *J Stud Alcohol* 1982;43:927–938.

20
The Elderly

KATHERINE HESSE and JOAN SAVITSKY

There is an increased need for primary care physicians to address alcohol use and abuse in the aged population in the United States, in part because of the dramatic expansion of this age group. A number of unique issues arise when evaluating the aging population for alcohol-related problems: (1) the usual screening criteria are not entirely appropriate for this age group, leading to underidentification and misdiagnosis, (2) the impact of alcohol on the older individual may be more intense due both to physiologic changes associated with normal aging and the frequency of acute and chronic medical problems, and (3) the cognitive deterioration that may accompany the chronic use of alcohol can further compromise functional capacity in the elderly.

Epidemiology

Several common themes emerge from studies on the incidence and prevalence of alcohol use and problem drinking in the elderly despite the wide variety of settings, such as communities, housing projects, general and psychiatric hospitals, and rehabilitation agencies.[1-5] Most find that alcohol consumption in the United States peaks under the age of 50 and then declines with age.[2,6] Fewer than 10% of men in their 70s are thought to be heavy drinkers. Abstinence is the most common drinking pattern for older women, and heavy drinking is seen in less than 2% of elderly women. Probably between 2% and 10% of those over 60 suffer from problems related to alcohol use.[7] It is estimated that 10% of all alcoholics are over 60,[8,9] and in some general hospitals and psychiatric facilities, between 5% and 44% of elderly patients may have alcohol-related problems.[10]

There are several hypotheses for the changes in drinking habits seen with aging, but these explanations require further study. Financial and lifestyle changes associated with retirement may decrease the availability of alcohol. The physiologic effects of aging and medical problems may interfere with the pleasurable effects of drinking. The current geriatric population may use alcohol at a lower rate because they lived through Prohibition and the Depression of the 1930s and never became heavy drinkers. Heavy drinkers may die at a younger age, leaving behind those with more moderate drinking habits.

Natural History

The elderly manifest two common patterns of alcohol abuse: the early-onset drinker who has grown old and the late-onset drinker who drinks in response to stresses associated with aging. Early-onset abusers comprise about two thirds of older drinkers.[9,11-13] They begin with heavy use of alcohol early in life (from the teens to the 40s) and continue either constantly or intermittently with advancing age, carrying into old age the social, psychologic, and medical problems associated with long-term alcohol abuse. Because chronic alcoholics have significant medical disease and a higher mortality rate than nonalcoholics, many enter the last years of their lives as they turn 65.[14,15] These patients are encountered frequently in institutional settings, especially acute care hospitals. Physicians often concentrate on treating such patients medically and do not attempt to alter the alcohol-related, self-destructive behavior.

In contrast, the natural history of the late-onset alcoholic may be more benign, with a better prognosis for stopping drinking.[16-19] Late-onset alcoholics may experience a reactive form of alcohol abuse.[20] Many losses are associated with the aging process, depression may follow, and alcohol abuse is one response to depression. Precipitants may include loneliness, poor health, retirement, and grief. If the cause of the problem is identified and treated as depression, some clinicians believe that there is a meaningful recovery rate,[16] but this assertion has not been studied.

The natural history of certain elderly drinkers may result in the geriatric squalor syndrome, in which elderly people live in a setting of filth and chaos, rejecting all attempts to change their lifestyles.[21] Although antisocial behavior usually declines with age, some elderly alcoholics continue to experience legal difficulties related to public drunkenness and other minor offenses.[22-24]

Physiology

The physiologic changes associated with aging may affect the absorption, peak blood level, and metabolism of alcohol. In one of few physiologic studies, Vestal et al found that older men achieved a higher peak blood alcohol concentration following intravenous administration of alcohol than did younger men.[25] Aging may also alter the acute and chronic effects of alcohol on the various organ systems. However, there is little experimental evidence addressing these concerns in human subjects.

The interaction among aging, the use of alcohol, and cognitive impairment poses three distinct questions. Does the chronic use of alcohol produce specific cognitive defects identical to those found in normal aging? Are older drinkers more susceptible than younger drinkers to the cognitive impairment associated with the use of alcohol? Does the chronic use of alcohol increase the risk for dementia?

Numerous researchers have attempted to compare the cognitive changes seen with normal aging with those seen in chronic drinkers. On neuropsychologic testing, younger heavy drinkers have many of the same impairments as normal, healthy elderly people.[27-29] This has led researchers to propose the hypothesis of premature aging: alcohol accelerates the changes in cognitive and neurophysiologic testing seen with normal aging. However, other data contradict the premature aging hypothesis.[30-32]

Is the aging brain more sensitive to alcohol than the brain of a younger person? Speculation exists that older nonalcoholic subjects may be more sensitive to the acute effects of alcohol.[33] Moderate social drinking by older people may result in chronic cognitive deficits.[34] Older late-onset heavy drinkers may develop cognitive impairments that are more significant than those manifested by younger drinkers who consume the same amount of alcohol over the same period of time.[32]

Dementia is a global impairment of brain function in which memory, intellect, language, personality, and visual-perceptual capacities fail progressively over time and interfere with functional capabilities. It is a disease process seen with increasing frequency with advancing age, but it is not a result of normal aging. Alcoholics have a higher than expected risk of both cerebral atrophy and dementia, independent of age.[11,12,35-37] The duration of drinking and amount of alcohol used combined with medical problems, such as repeated head trauma and liver disease, may contribute to this increased risk.[37] Alcohol itself, however, may not be the direct cause of the cognitive impairment.[38] This process may also incorporate the alcohol-related Wernicke-Korsakoff dementia of thiamine deficiency, which can produce a continuum of amnestic deficits.[39] It is not clear whether there is an increased risk of true Alzheimer's dementia among alcoholics.[35]

Diagnosis

The drinking behavior of young and middle-aged males is the basis for most diagnostic criteria and screening tools for alcoholism. The described patterns of drinking and alcohol-related problems do not consistently identify behaviors and problems seen in older alcoholics. For example, screening instruments typically examine the individual's social life for evidence that it is affected by drinking. Has the person lost a job? Is the home life disrupted? Have there been encounters with the law for drunken driving or brawling? Elderly alcoholics are often retired from active employment and may be socially isolated, without frequent family contacts. They may have curtailed their driving activities and are unlikely to engage in physical conflict.

Another standard method for assessing drinking behavior is to quantify the amount of alcohol used. However, there is no consensus on acceptable levels of alcohol consumption for the aged person. A number of factors associated with the aging process modify the significance of simple quantification of alcohol intake. An elderly, retired businessman who habitually takes two cocktails before dinner may experience confusion with this amount of alcohol as he develops mild cognitive impairment due to early Alzheimer-type dementia. A frail elderly woman who is unsteady on her feet may no longer safely enjoy an occasional glass of sherry.

Alcohol has a variety of deleterious physical effects, often insignificant in the young, that can aggravate changes in the normal aging process and problems associated with acute or chronic disease in the elderly. Balance and coordination are affected. Confusion may develop or worsen. The regulation of temperature may be impaired, increasing the age-related risk of hypothermia. The diuretic effect of alcohol may be significant in the frail elderly. Arrhythmias and impaired left ventricular function are potential cardiac side effects.[40,41]

Many older people take one or more medications that present additional hazards when used with alcohol. Used acutely or chronically, alcohol modifies the metabolism of certain drugs so that their effect becomes unpredictable.[10,42,43] In addition, because of the confusional state produced by alcohol, patients may be unable to take their medication appropriately, and drugs may combine with alcohol to cause further confusion. Alcohol may enhance effects or side effects of medication, such as the vasodilation produced by nitrates. Chloral hydrate and the sulfonylureas occasionally produce a disulfiram-like reaction when taken with alcohol.[43,44] Alcohol is especially dangerous in the elderly patient taking warfarin derivatives because of its direct effect on drug metabolism, as well as the increased risk of falls and gastrointestinal bleeding.

Physicians all too often evaluate and treat medical problems in the elderly without recognizing their relation to alcohol. Signs, symptoms, and laboratory abnormalities (nonspecific but suspicious for alcoholism in a healthy younger population) are attributed either to the normal aging process or to underlying medical problems in older patients. Confusion, disturbances in sleep, anxiety, depression, noncompliance, tremors, gait abnormalities, falls, multiple fractures, osteoporosis, gastrointestinal complaints, malnutrition, congestive heart failure, and palpitations are all common in the nonalcoholic older person but may also be due to, or aggravated by, the use of alcohol.[10,44,45] Similarly, laboratory findings, such as liver function abnormalities, anemia, macrocytosis, platelet disorders, bleeding abnormalities, vitamin deficiencies, and hyperuricemia, can be due either to commonly encountered medical problems in the elderly or to the use of alcohol. Finally, alcohol withdrawal is commonly overlooked during hospitalization of an elderly patient because transient confusion is so common in this population.

Recognition of an alcohol-related problem requires the physician first to consider the diagnosis in an elderly person, even when apparent use is minimal and answers to screening questions are negative. The use of alcohol should be ruled out when neuropsychiatric symptoms, such as depression, confusion, and abnormal behavior, occur. Functional problems that interfere with daily life, such as poor grooming, malnutrition, frequent falls, and incontinence, may provide clues to problems with alcohol, as may social difficulties, such as isolation and estrangement from family.[10,45] In the frail or otherwise compromised elderly patient, any use of alcohol may be too much.

Treatment

Pessimism about the usefulness of treating the elderly problem drinker may exclude older drinkers from treatment programs.[46-49] The limited research available, however, suggests that older drinkers have as favorable a response to treatment as younger alcoholics,[1,50] and the elderly may benefit from a broader range of services than younger alcoholics.[1,51] As with other populations, the elderly hold strong beliefs about the stigma of alcohol abuse. Once having acknowledged the drinking problem, the frail elderly may have additional difficulty in using community treatment outreach programs due to physical and mental limitations. For those with functional problems, transportation, homemaker assistance, home-delivered meals, or home visits may help them engage in treatment.

Because of the risk of complications in the elderly with medical problems, those who require detoxification should be monitored in an inpatient setting. When there is no medical problem and a responsible person is in the home to supervise, mild withdrawal can be treated at home with close medical follow-up.

During the withdrawal process, many geriatricians prefer to use short-acting benzodiazepines, such as oxazepam, to avoid accumulation of drug and overmedication.[52,53,54] The dose must be titrated based on close clinical observation, and caution must be taken when using short-acting drugs to avoid periods of undermedication. The major risks during withdrawal include oversedation and aspiration, tachycardia with cardiovascular consequences, and delirium with agitation resulting in trauma. Thiamine administration and screening for dietary deficiencies (such as folate, vitamin B_{12}, and magnesium) are advised. Older patients may take longer to complete the withdrawal process, and the subacute confusional state may last for weeks, making rehabilitation during that period difficult. Elderly people who have abused alcohol may also be polydrug abusers, and signs and symptoms of sedative, barbiturate, tranquilizer, or narcotic abuse complicate the detoxification process. Prolonged withdrawal symptoms may be due to concurrent use of prescription drugs, such as the long-acting benzodiazepines.[10,52,53,54] It is important to remember that improvements in mental functioning may not occur until many weeks after detoxification.

After detoxification, the elderly drinker requires an interdisciplinary evaluation to assess medical, psychologic, and social problems. Failing health and functional limitations may contribute to depression associated with alcohol abuse in the older drinker. Therefore, careful attention should be paid to treating correctable medical conditions and maximizing functional capacities. A clinical depression resulting from the patient's drinking may resolve with sobriety, but it is important to undertake a full psychologic assessment, searching for emotional stresses that may have led to reactive drinking. Other psychiatric and cognitive problems that may interfere with rehabilitation must be identified.

Inpatient rehabilitation programs often accept older patients, but elders may feel left out of the general milieu of the program, and solutions specific to their needs are often overlooked. These problems can be overcome by involving family members in the therapeutic efforts[1,55,56] addressing issues related to aging and offering an opportunity for socialization.[1,55–57] The backbone of outpatient treatment, Alcoholics Anonymous, is often an excellent resource, since it provides the social support network frequently lacking in the life of the older alcoholic. Many frail elderly, however, may be reticent to participate in such programs unless the group includes other older participants.

Many clinicians are reluctant to consider pharmacologic treatments of alcohol abuse for older patients, but medically stable elderly patients with good cognitive function and motivation may be candidates for disulfiram therapy, taking into account the usual contraindications (Chap. 8). Antidepressants are effective with some late-onset drinkers.[17] Medications with the lowest risk of anticholinergic, sedating, or orthostatic side effects should be prescribed, such as desipramine, nortriptyline, and trazodone.[52,53,54] Initial doses should be low (less than 50% of the usual adult starting dose) and increased slowly to full therapeutic dosage. Patients should receive an adequate trial of at least 8 to 12 weeks at therapeutic doses. Benzodiazepines or sedative hypnotics taken chronically substitute one dependence for another and should be avoided.

The popular assertion that moderate use of alcohol in healthy, older persons lifts the spirits, increases sociability, and, according to some, improves mental function in socially conducive settings requires further study. Some advocate the use of alcohol as a social stimulant in nursing home settings.[58] However, the marked variation in the health of nursing home residents and in their tolerance to alcohol necessitates an evaluation for each individual.

Alcohol use in the elderly presents numerous problems which are too often attributed by physicians to the aging process. The metabolism of alcohol in the normal elder and the specific risks of the frail elder who uses alcohol need careful attention. There is currently no consensus about recommendations for alcohol use in the aging individual. Maintaining a high level of suspicion, questioning about alcohol use persistently, and utilizing interdisciplinary community resources can make the care of an older problem drinker more appropriate and effective.

References

1. Gomberg ESL: Alcohol use and alcohol problems among the elderly, in *Alcohol and Health, Special Population Issues*. Monograph No. 4. Rockville, Md, National Institute on Alcohol Abuse and Alcoholism, 1982:263–290.
2. Barnes GM: Alcohol use among older persons: Findings from a western New York state general population survey. *J Am Geriatr Soc* 1979,27:244–250.

3. Room R: Drinking patterns in large US cities; A comparison of San Francisco and national samples. *Q J Stud Alcohol* 1972;6(suppl):28–59.
4. Schuckit MA, Miller PL: Alcoholism in elderly men: A survey of a general medical ward. *Ann NY Acad Sci* 1976;273:558–571.
5. Kramer M: *Patients in State and County Mental Hospitals*. Public Health Service Publication No 1921. Chevy Chase, Md, National Institute of Mental Health, 1979.
6. Cahalan D, Cisin IH, Crosley HM: *American Drinking Practices: A National Study of Drinking Behavior and Attitudes*. Monograph No. 6. New Brunswick, NJ, Rutgers Center of Alcohol Studies, 1969.
7. Schuckit MA, Pastore PA: The elderly as a unique population: Alcoholism. *Alcoholism Clin Exp Res* 1978;2:31–38.
8. Schuckit MA: Geriatric alcoholism and drug abuse. *Gerontologist* 1977;17:168–174.
9. Rosen AJ, Blatt MM: Alcohol excess in the elderly. *Q J Stud Alcohol* 1971;32:53–59.
10. Atkinson RM, Kofoed LL: Alcohol and drug abuse in old age, in Cassel CK, Walsh JR (eds): *Geriatric Medicine*. New York, Springer Verlag, 1984, vol 2, *Fundamentals of Geriatric Care*, pp 219–235.
11. Simon A, Epstein LJ, Reynolds L: Alcoholism in geriatric mentally ill. *Geriatrics* 1968;23:125–131.
12. Gaitz CM, Baer PE: Characteristics of elderly patients with alcoholism. *Arch Gen Psychiatry* 1971;24:372–378.
13. Atkinson R, Kofoed LL: Alcohol and drug abuse in old age: A clinical perspective. *Substance and alcohol actions/misuse*. 1982;3:353–368.
14. Drew LRH: Alcoholism as a self-limiting disease. *Q J Stud Alcohol* 1960;29:956–967.
15. deLindt J, Schmidt W: Alcoholism and mortality, in Kissen B, Begleiter H (eds): *Social Aspects of Alcoholism*. New York, Plenum, 1976, pp 275–305.
16. Zimberg S: The elderly alcoholic. *Gerontologist* 1974;14:221–224.
17. Zimberg S: Two types of problem drinkers: Both can be managed. *Geriatrics* 1974;29:135–139.
18. Pascarelli EF: Drug dependence: An age-old problem compounded by old age. *Geriatrics* 1974;29:109–115.
19. Wilkenson P: Alcoholism in the aged. *J Geriatr* 1971;34:59–64.
20. Hartford JT, Theinhaus OJ: Psychiatric aspects of alcoholism in geriatric patients, in Hartford JT, Samorajski T (eds): *Alcoholism in the Elderly.* New York, Raven Press, 1984, pp 253–261.
21. Kafetz K, Cox M: Alcohol excess and the senile squalor syndrome. *J Am Geriatr Soc* 1982;30:706.
22. Epstein LJ, Mills C, Simon A: Antisocial behavior of the elderly. *Comp Psychiatry* 1970;11:36–42.
23. Zax M, Gardner EA, Hart WT: Public intoxication in Rochester: A survey of individuals charged with public drunkenness during 1961. *Q J Stud Alcohol* 1964;25:669–678.
24. Zung BJ: Sociodemographic correlates of problem drinking among DWI offenders. *J Stud Alcohol* 1979;40:1064–1072.
25. Vestal RE, McGuire EA, Tobin JD, et al: Aging and ethanol metabolism in man. *Clin Pharmacol Ther* 1977;21:343–354.
26. Katzman R, Terry R: Normal aging of the nervous system, in Katzman R, Terry R (eds): *The Neurology of Aging*. Philadelphia, FA Davis, 1983, pp 15–57.

27. Ryan C, Butters N: Learning and memory impairments in young and old alcoholics: Evidence for the premature aging hypothesis. *Alcoholism Clin Exp Res* 1980;4:288–293.
28. Bradt J, Butters N, Ryan C, Bayog R: Cognitive loss and recovery in long-term alcohol abuse. *Arch Gen Psychiatry* 1983;40:435–442.
29. Becker JT, Butters N, Herman A, D'Angelo N: A comparison of the effects of long-term alcohol abuse and aging on the performance of verbal and nonverbal divided attention tasks. *Alcoholism Clin Exp Res* 1983;7:213–219.
30. Porjesz B, Begleiter H, Samuelly I: Cognitive deficits in chronic alcoholics and elderly subjects assessed by evoked brain potentials. *Acta Psychiatr Scand* 1980;62(suppl 286):15–29.
31. Grant I, Adams K, Reed R: Aging, abstinence and medical risk factors in the prediction of neuropsychological deficit among long-term alcoholics. *Arch Gen Psychiatry* 1984;41:710–718.
32. Ryan C: Alcoholism and premature aging: A neuropsychological perspective. *Alcoholism Clin Exp Res* 1982;6:22–30.
33. Ritzmann RF, Melchior CL: Age and development of tolerance to and physical dependence on alcohol, in Hartford JT, Samorajski T (eds): *Alcoholism in the Elderly.* New York, Raven Press, 1984, pp 117–137.
34. Parker ES, Noble EP: Alcohol and the aging process in social drinkers. *J Stud Alcohol* 1980;41:170–178.
35. Meyer JS, Largen JW, Shaw T, et al: Interactions of normal aging, senile dementia, multiinfarct dementia, and alcoholism in the elderly, in Hartford JT, Samorajski T (eds): *Alcoholism and the Elderly.* New York, Raven Press, 1984, pp 227–251.
36. William JD, Ray CG, Overall JE: Mental aging and organicity in an alcoholic population. *J Consult Clin Psychol* 1973;41:392–396.
37. Carlen PL, Wilkenson DA, Wortzman G, et al: Cerebral atrophy and functional deficits in alcoholism without clinically apparent liver disease. *Neurology* 1981;31:377–385.
38. Adams RD, Victor M: *Principles of Neurology.* New York, McGraw Hill, 1981, pp 757–758.
39. Ryan C, Butters N, Montgomery K, et al: Memory deficits in chronic alcoholics: Continuities between the "intact" alcoholic and the alcoholic Korsakoff patient, in Begleiter H (ed): *Biologic Effects of Alcohol.* New York, Plenum, 1980, pp 701–718.
40. Gambert SR, Newton M, Duthie EH: Medical issues in alcoholism in the elderly, in Hartford JT, Samorajski T (eds): *Alcoholism and the Elderly.* New York, Raven Press, 1984, pp 175–191.
41. Mishara BL, Kastenbaum R: *Alcohol and Old Age.* New York, Grune & Stratton. 1980, pp 13–40.
42. Seixas FA: Drug/alcohol interactions: avert potential dangers. *Geriatrics* 1979;34:89–102.
43. Gerbino PP: Complications of alcohol use combined with drug therapy in the elderly. *J Am Geriatr Soc* 1982;30(suppl):S88–S93.
44. Hartford T, Samorajski T: Alcoholism in the geriatric populations. *J Am Geriatr Soc* 1982;30:18–24.
45. Wattis JP: Alcohol problems in the elderly. *J Am Geriatr Soc* 1981;29:131–134.
46. Knox WJ: Attitudes of psychiatrists and psychologists toward alcoholics. *Am J Psychol* 1971;127:1675–1729.

47. Kola LA, Kosberg JI, Joyce K: The alcoholic elderly client: Assessment of policies and practices in service providers. *Gerontologist* 1984;24:519–521.
48. Bozzetti LP, MacMurray JP: Drug misuse among the elderly: A hidden menace. *Psychiatr Ann* 1971;7:95–107.
49. Meyers AR, Hingson R, Mucatel M, Goldman E: Social and psychologic correlates of problem drinking in old age. *J Am Geriatr Soc* 1982;30:452–456.
50. Mishara BL, Kastenbaum R: *Alcohol and Old Age*. New York, Grune & Stratton, 1980, pp 85–102.
51. Schuckit MA: A clinical review of alcohol, alcoholism and the elderly patient. *J Clin Psychiatr* 1982;43:396–399.
52. Salzman C: A primer on geriatric psychopharmacology. *Am J Psychiatry* 1982;139:67–74.
53. Thompson TL,Moran MG, Nies AS: Psychotropic drug use in the elderly, Part I. *N Engl J Med* 1983;308:134–138.
54. Thompson TL, Moran MG, Nies AS: Psychotropic drug use in the elderly, Part II. *N Engl J Med.* 1983;308:194–199.
55. Rathbone-McCuan E, Triegaardt J: The older alcoholic and the family. *Alcohol Health Research World* 1976;3:7–12.
56. Older problem drinkers. *Alcohol Health Research World* 1975;3:12–17.
57. Hall EP: Substance abuse in the aging, in Bennett G, Vourakis C, Woolf DS (eds): *Substance Abuse: Pharmacologic, Developmental and Clinical Perspectives*. New York, John Wiley & Sons, 1983, pp 192–205.
58. Mishara BL, Kastenbaum R: *Alcohol and Old Age*. New York, Grune & Stratton, 1980, pp 127–162.

21
Women and Alcohol Abuse

ANDREA HALLIDAY and BOOKER BUSH

According to a Gallup Poll, the number of women in the United States who drink alcohol has increased from 45% to 66% over the last 40 years.[1] Claims that the number of women alcohol abusers increased dramatically during this period may reflect shifts in social and political perspective rather than real changes.[2,3] However, recent evidence suggests that heavy drinking is on the rise among young, employed women.[4] Whether or not the pattern of drinking among women is converging with the pattern of male drinking, it is clear that a smaller percentage of female problem drinkers enter treatment for alcohol abuse compared to male problem drinkers.[2] Because society considers it less acceptable for a woman to be a heavy drinker than a man, a woman's drinking problem is often hidden or ignored by families, police, friends, and employers. These attitudes delay or prevent women from receiving treatment.[1,3,5,6]

Although alcohol abuse in women is a hidden problem, the problem is significant. Surveys in the community indicate that 5% of women drink heavily (three to five drinks a day),[7] but surveys of gynecology practices show that 12% to 16% of patients are heavy drinkers.[8,9] Because of the bias of underreporting, these surveys may actually underestimate the degree of problem drinking among women.

Etiology

The etiology of alcoholism in women is particularly difficult to define because of the paucity of good longitudinal data. Both heredity and environment may predispose women to abuse alcohol, and the presence of alcoholism in a sibling, parent, spouse, lover, or even among friends may be a significant risk factor.[1,2,5,6] Vaillant's 30-year prospective study in men confirms the importance of family history (heredity and environment) in the development of alcoholism,[10] but no studies to date have addressed whether women are more susceptible than men to environmental influences in the development of the disease.

Factors reflecting women's unique physiology, such as menopause, postpartum depression, and severe premenstrual changes in mood, have all been mentioned as possible precipitants for alcohol abuse in women, but clear documentation is lacking.[6,8,9] Clinical data from programs treating women for alcohol abuse show a 45% to 70% prevalence of rape, incest, or both in their clients, suggesting a possible role for early sexual abuse as a precipitant for alcohol abuse. This correlation has not been examined prospectively.[3,5]

Natural History

Women begin to abuse alcohol at a later age than men, usually in their late 20s or early 30s, but they enter alcohol treatment programs and develop the physical manifestations of alcoholism at an average age of 40 to 50 years, the same as for men.[6,11] This phenomenon of rapid progression from abusive drinking to late-stage alcoholism is referred to as "telescoping."

In most studies that describe the development of physical complications of alcoholism, the average duration of heavy drinking was shorter for women than for men. Statistically significant differences in rates of development have been found for ulcer surgery, gastrointestinal hemorrhage, fatty liver, hypertension, obesity, anemia, and malnutrition. In these surveys, women had been alcoholic for 14 years, whereas the duration of alcoholism for men was 20 years.[12,13]

The mortality rate attributable to alcoholism is greater in women. Whereas the death rate among male alcoholics is two to four times that of men in the general population, the death rate for alcoholic women is 2.7 to seven times that of women in the general population.[12,13] This difference, of course, may reflect only the fact that alcoholism in women is not detected until the disease is advanced.

The prevalence of alcoholism and its medical complications vary among subpopulations of alcoholic women. The small amount of empiric data available suggests that certain groups of women are at very high risk. The 1975 cirrhosis death rate among Native American women was approximately 8%. The corresponding figures for black and white women were 2.6% and 1.7%, respectively. No data were reported for other ethnic minorities.[14] A study comparing the psychologic adjustment of lesbians and female heterosexuals found no significant difference in rates of affective disorders, neuroses, and personality disturbances. However, the presence of alcoholism in the lesbian population was seven times higher than in the heterosexual population.[15]

Diagnostic Considerations

The information required to confirm a diagnosis of alcoholism or alcohol abuse in women is the same as that for men. There may be some important differences, though, in complaints. For women, the complaint will often be one or more of a wide range of symptoms, including depression, anxiety, sleeplessness, lethargy, stomach problems, and injuries from accidents or physical abuse.[6,16] Obstetric and gynecologic disorders may give clues to underlying alcohol abuse. Alcoholic women compared with nonalcoholic controls report an increased incidence of infertility, miscarriage, postpartum depression, irregular menstrual cycles, and amenorrhea.[8,9,13] A twofold increase in alcoholism and alcohol abuse in women seeking care for premenstrual syndrome was found as compared with women seeking periodic gynecologic care.[8]

A diagnosis based on the quantity of alcohol consumed may be misleading because women generally need to consume less alcohol than men to feel both its positive and negative effects. The blood alcohol levels from a given amount of alcohol are greater in women than in men due to women's lighter weights and lower ratio of lean body mass to adipose tissue. Women who use oral contraceptives metabolize ethanol significantly more slowly than women not using this type of contraceptive. Furthermore, in the premenstrual phase, women absorb alcohol more quickly and completely than in the postmenstrual phase.[17] The clinical significance of these facts is unclear.

Alcohol abuse has been called the "hidden" or "invisible" problem in women. Many women who abuse alcohol do so at home and alone. Female problem drinkers are less likely than male problem drinkers to report difficulties with work, the law, or violent behavior. They are more inclined to report problems with their relationships and children as a result of drinking.[5,6,11,18] Drinking by oneself suggests a nonsocial use of alcohol. Eliciting this history when there is other evidence suggestive of alcohol abuse may confirm the diagnosis.

Treatment

Although the principles of treatment are similar for men and women, there are several issues specific to women alcoholics that must be considered in establishing a treatment plan. In addition to a thorough history and physical examination to identify potential alcohol withdrawal or other problems that require medical intervention, a complete history of drug use should be taken. A majority of alcoholic women abuse other drugs, usually prescribed sedative hypnotic medications rather than illicit drugs.[6,11,16] Therapy should center on detoxification, education, and supportive care. Women alcoholics, like their male counterparts, suffer from low self-esteem, feelings of inadequacy, and extreme guilt.[1,3,5,6] However, unlike men, the social roles of many alcoholic women tend to reinforce a devalued self-image. For instance, alcoholic women are more likely than nonalcoholic women to have alcoholic husbands or lovers and be at increased risk for domestic violence.[5,19,20] Frequently, women alcoholics are incest survivors, victims of child or spouse abuse, rape victims, or daughters of alcoholic parents.[1,3,5,6,11] Women, alcoholic or not, perceive themselves as having more dependency needs, less control over their lives, and less need to control others.[19]

Alcoholism treatment programs for women can address these issues directly. Single-sex therapy groups with female staff members serving as role models provide a safe environment in which to work on questions of self-esteem and assertiveness. Women are more willing to discuss sensitive issues, such as sexual abuse, in all-female support groups.[5] Peer groups of alcoholic mothers can provide the opportunity to express guilt feelings about the effects of alcoholism on their children.[5]

To be truly effective, a treatment program for alcoholic women must address their practical needs as well. In a New Jersey drug and alcohol program, 96% of the women interviewed stated that lack of job training was a major concern.[1] A 1977 study by the National Institute for Alcoholism and Alcohol Abuse showed that only 30% of the 60,000 women entering treatment were employed and that the mean household income was $7,000.[1]

The disadvantaged position of alcoholic women in society-at-large has significant implications for their access to care. Many are unable to afford appropriate treatment. The lack of suitable child care, particularly for residential programs, is a major barrier.[1,3,5] Women are less likely than men to receive support from family and friends for entering treatment.[16] A common belief among health care professionals is that women do less well in treatment than men,[4] despite the fact that there is no good evidence to support this contention.[21] The problems experienced by women in general are compounded for women from ethnic minorities and lesbians. Not only do these groups have higher rates of alcoholism and its complications,[1,14,15] but the negative attitudes of caregivers have prevented them from seeking needed treatment.[1,3,5]

In formulating a treatment plan with an alcoholic woman patient, the physician must assess the patient's special needs and discuss openly the advantages and limitations of different treatment options. Although there is no evidence currently that women alcoholics respond better to female therapists, many patients prefer to work with a counselor of the same sex.[5] Culture-specific programs may be necessary to attract and keep minority women in treatment; however, this hypothesis has not been tested.[14] Given the paucity of services for women, whether in all-women's programs or coeducational centers, the physician may need to take an active role in ensuring that the patient receives adequate treatment for her alcoholism.

Female alcoholism is not a qualitatively different syndrome from male alcoholism, and the self-destructive effects of alcoholism supersede any gender differences. However, because the social roles of men and women differ, female alcoholism encompasses a unique set of issues. These issues must be addressed to engage and keep women in treatment.

References

1. Sandmaier M: *The Invisible Alcoholics: Women and Alcohol in America*. New York, McGraw-Hill, 1980.
2. Wilsnack SC, Wilsnack RW, Klassen AD: Drinking and drinking problems among women in a US national survey. *Alcohol Health Res World* 1984/5;15:3–13.

3. Beckman LJ, Amaro H: Patterns of women's use of alcohol treatment agencies, in Wilsnack SC, Beck LJ (eds): *Alcohol Problems in Women*. New York, The Guilford Press, 1983.
4. Fillmore KM: When angels fall: Women's drinking as cultural preoccupation and as reality, in Wilsnack SC, Beck LJ (eds): *Alcohol Problems in Women*. New York, The Guilford Press, 1983.
5. Hamilton G, Volpe J: How women recover: Experience and research observations. *Alcohol Health Res World* 1982/3;7:28–39.
6. Schuckit MA, Morrisey ER: Alcoholism in women: Some clinical and social perspectives with an emphasis on possible subtypes, in Greenblatt M, Schuckit MA (eds): *Alcoholism Problems in Women and Children*. New York, Grune & Stratton, 1976, pp 5–36.
7. Armor DJ, Polich JM, Stambul HB: *Alcoholism and Treatment*. New York, Wiley and Jones, 1978.
8. Halliday A, Bush B, Cleary P, et al: Alcohol abuse in women seeking gynecologic care. *Obstet Gynecol* 1986;68(3):322–326.
9. Russell M, Bigler L: Screening for alcohol-related problems in an outpatient obstetric-gynecologic clinic. *Am J Obstet Gynecol* 1979;134:4–12.
10. Vaillant GE: *The Natural History of Alcoholism: Causes, Patterns, and Paths to Recovery*. Cambridge, Mass, Harvard University Press, 1983.
11. Mulford HA: Women and men problem drinkers: Sex differences in patients served by Iowa's community alcoholism centers. *J Stud Alcohol* 1977;38:1624–1639.
12. Ashley MJ, Olin JS, Harding le Riche W, et al: Morbidity in alcoholics: Evidence for accelerated development of physical disease in women. *Arch Intern Med* 1977;137:883–887.
13. Hill SY: Biological consequences of alcoholism and alcohol-related problems among women, in *Alcohol and Health: Special Population Issues*. Monograph No 4. Rockville, Md, DHHS, 1982:43–76.
14. Leland J: Alcohol use and abuse in ethnic minority women, in Wilsnack SC, Beck LJ (eds): *Alcohol Problems in Women*. New York, The Guilford Press, 1983.
15. Saghir MT, Robins E, Walbram B, Gentry KA: Homosexuality. IV. Psychiatric disorders and disability in the female homosexual. *Am J Psychiatry* 1970;127:147–154.
16. Schuckit MA, Morrisey MA: Drug abuse among alcoholic women. *Am J Psychiatry 1979;136:607*–611.
17. Jones BM, Jones MK: Women and alcohol: Intoxication, metabolism, and the menstrual cycle, in Greenblatt M, Schuckit MA (eds): *Alcoholism Problems in Women and Children*. New York, Grune & Stratton, 1976, pp 103–136.
18. Celentano DD, McQueen DV, Chee E: Substance abuse by women: A review of the epidemiologic literature. *J Chronic Dis* 1980;33:383–394.
19. Frieze IH, Schafer PC: Alcohol use and marital violence: Female and male differences in reactions to alcohol, in Wilsnack SC, Beck LJ (eds): *Alcohol Problems in Women*. New York, The Guilford Press, 1983.
20. Williams CN, Klerman LV: Female alcohol abuse: Its effects on the family, in Wilsnack SC, Beck LJ (eds): *Alcohol Problems in Women*. New York. The Guilford Press, 1983.
21. Vannicelli M: Treatment outcome of alcoholic women: The state of the art in relation to sex bias and expectancy effects, in Wilsnack SC, Beck LJ (eds): *Alcohol Problems in Women*. New York, The Guilford Press, 1983.

22
The Adolescent Drinker

MARGARET BEAN-BAYOG

Mary is 20 years old, pretty, popular, and an honors graduate of a prestigious girls' college. She is seen on her second admission for detoxification from alcohol. During five years of problem drinking followed by three years of addictive alcoholism, she has been seen by seven physicians. Not one had diagnosed or treated her. She continues to deny her alcoholism, even though she has experienced blackouts increasing in frequency from one every six months at age 13 to every two weeks at age 18 and has been involved in two car accidents. She is aware of her family's concern over her frequent drunkenness and has low self-esteem. Her relationships with nondrinking peers have slowly deteriorated, as she began to prefer heavy drinking and drug-using companions. Six months before her most recent admission, morning withdrawal sickness led to tardiness and difficulty performing her job, but she still continued the facade that her drunkenness was part of a carefree, party lifestyle.

None of her physicians believed that this appealing young person belonged in the diagnostic category of alcoholism. Even if they had been convinced, their training failed to equip them with the skills and courage needed to deal with it.

A young person between the ages of 12 and 20 with a drinking problem poses a particular challenge for the physician. The difficulties encountered when working with adult alcoholics are intensified when found in adolescents.

Epidemiology

Unfortunately, teenage drinking problems and alcoholism are becoming increasingly common, while rates of other drug use have declined.[1] Rachal et al's 1978 survey of youthful drinking practices conducted for the National Institute on Alcohol Abuse and Alcoholism found that nearly one third of 4,918 high school students reported moderately heavy drinking, and 15% were drinking to drunkenness (defined as five drinks per occasion) at least once a week. Even when young students (grades 7 to 9) were included, more than 10% of the teenagers classified themselves in the heaviest category.[2] Girls and very young teenagers are now drinking at rates approaching those of adult males.[3] All these data on rates of teenage drinking exceed the prevalence rates of drinking problems of adults. In other words, teenagers in the United States are drinking more than adults, even though it is illegal. This disturbing fact may be somewhat obscured by the types of problems teenagers experience as a result of drinking.

Characteristics

Physical addiction and symptoms of withdrawal do occur in adolescents but with less frequency than in adults. Social problems of the magnitude of job loss and marital strain are less common. Parents may protest and punish teenage drinking, but they rarely withdraw food and shelter. Cirrhosis of the liver, a complication of adult alcoholism, is rarely seen in teenagers, since it has not had time to develop.

Although adolescents escape problems common in adults, an alarming proportion suffer serious consequences as a result of drinking. Alcohol-related accidents are the number one cause of deaths. Ten thousand people aged 16 to 24 are killed every year, and many more are maimed.[4] Less dramatic, but far more frequent and insidious, are the developmental, psychologic, and social consequences of teenage alcohol abuse. At such a crucial time in their development, adolescents' experience and coping skills are not equal to the challenge. Regular, heavy use of any drug as a coping mechanism compromises psychologic growth and maturity. In addition to the normal, rapidly shifting stresses of adolescence, heavy drinking adds turmoil and trauma.[5] All this occurs at a time when adolescents should long for independence, begin to seek their adult identity, and start to acquire social skills. Problem drinking adolescents often remain financially dependent on parents, and relationships with peers remain shallow, leading to low self-esteem and depression.[6]

Another group of symptoms results from the intoxicated state: a high blood-alcohol level depresses the central nervous system and engenders impaired coordination and judgment. A teenager may describe symptoms, such as difficulty in school with missed classes or late assignments, memory blackouts, depression, thoughts of suicide and even attempts, family disruption, disorderly behavior, destruction of property, violence, or even homicide. This nonsocial drinking is associated with sexual promiscuity, poor work performance, social immaturity, lack of hobbies and interests, defensiveness, sensitivity, and isolation. Some of these symptoms may be physiologically based. The high schooler who drinks a six-pack of beer will show not only acute impairment but up to 72 hours later continues to have diminished short-term memory and decreased ability to process cognitive information.[7]

The social situation of the teenage drinker may contribute to additional difficulties. A high proportion of these teenagers are living with a family member, usually a parent, who is alcoholic or chemically dependent, often undiagnosed. The adolescent problem drinker has an increased risk of developing adult alcoholism. Donovan et al studied a cohort of college freshmen and followed them nine years later. Those students who were problem drinkers as freshmen were twice as likely to be adult problem drinkers as their nonproblem drinking classmates.[8]

Assessment

The diagnosis of alcoholism relies almost exclusively on history, but adolescents may be reluctant participants in the diagnostic process. They are financially secure and socially dependent and, therefore, experience very few consequences or losses due to drinking. Because of this genuine lack of experiential pain, adolescents have a hard time understanding why people around them are worried.[9] They see alcohol use as safe and enjoyable. They believe that adults, especially physicians, are judgmental authority figures bent on depriving them. Concern about labeling an adolescent with a stigmatizing diagnosis is valid. This is a sensitive time in identity formation, but it is important to clarify the diagnosis and not collude with the patient's denial.

The physician should be suspicious if anyone in the adolescent's immediate environs—family, school, court— raises a question about alcohol or drug use. In such cases, the diagnosis of dependence or abuse is highly likely. Other factors that should arouse suspicion are a family history of drinking or drug taking, use of minor tranquilizers, symptoms of family conflict, school failure, or depression. When the issue of drinking is raised, it is useful for the physician to ask questions about the adverse effects of drinking, such as "Does your drinking worry you? Has it caused trouble for you, such as conflicts with family, friends, teachers, or police? Does it make you sick or cause blackouts?" However, it may be easier to introduce the subject of drunkenness by questions about drinking patterns, "How often do you drink? When did you have your last drink? What was the purpose of taking a drink (to feel like one of the group, to feel adult, to drown your nervousness or sadness)?"[10] The questions used for adult diagnosis may be useful with some modifications. A version of the MAST with questions and scoring adapted for adolescents is shown in Table 22.1.

Because the adolescent may be unable to provide a good history, it is important to obtain additional information from others involved. Most parents, teachers, guidance counselors, and judges still view alcoholics as a skid row stereotype, and most cannot make the causal link between symptoms and drinking or drug use. However, they can give information about behavior. It is important to inquire about other drugs. It is rare to see an adolescent with a problem of abuse of only alcohol or only one drug.

Confronting the Patient

Once the diagnosis is made, the physician must share the information with the patient and family. Specific recommendations for treatment should be conveyed with an attitude of optimism. At this point, one often sees a sulky, uncooperative

TABLE 22.1. MAST adapted for use with adolescents.

	Yes	No
0. Do you enjoy a drink now and then?	0	
1. Do you feel you are a normal drinker? (By normal, we mean you drink less than or as much as most other people.)		2
2. Have you ever awakened the morning after some drinking the night before and found that you could not remember a part of the evening?	2	
3. Do either of your parents or any other near relative ever worry or complain about your drinking?	2	
4. Can you stop drinking without a struggle after one or two drinks?		2
5. Do you feel guilty about your drinking?	1	
6. Do friends and relatives think you are a normal drinker?		2
7. Are you able to stop drinking when you want to?		2
8. Have you ever attended a meeting of Alcoholics Anonymous (AA)?	5	
9. Have you gotten into physical fights when drinking?	1	
10. Has your drinking ever created problems between you and either your parents or another relative?	2	
11. Has either of your parents (or family member) ever gone to anyone for help about your drinking?	2	
12. Have you ever lost friends because of your drinking?	2	
13. Have you ever gotten into trouble at school or work because of drinking?	2	
14. Have you ever lost a job because of drinking?	2	
15. Have you ever neglected your school work, your obligations, your family, or your work for two or more days in a row because you were drinking?	2	
16. Do you drink before noon fairly often?	1	
17. Have you ever been told you have liver trouble? Cirrhosis?	2	
18. After heavy drinking have you ever had delirium tremens (DTs) or severe shaking or heard voices or seen things that really weren't there?	2[a]	
19. Have you ever gone to anyone for help because of drinking?	5	
20. Have you ever been in a hospital because of drinking?	5	
21. Have you ever been a patient in a psychiatric hospital or on a psychiatric ward of a general hospital where drinking was part of the problem that resulted in hospitalization?	2	

teenager who does not experience any personal threat from his drug use. One has to discover if this negativity is a result of alcoholic denial, the patient's failure to grasp the seriousness of the problem, a developmental preference for action over verbal abstractions, an assertion of a separate identity from adult authorities, or a result of recent drug taking. Whatever the source, the negative attitude must be faced if the adolescent is to be treated. Much of the resistance to treatment decreases if the adolescent agrees to undertake a trial of staying drug free. One way to deal with an adolescent's resistance is to meet with the adolescent and other important figures—parents, a teacher, or probation officer. The alcohol problem is presented, and the teenager is asked if he has tried to stop, has reason to stop, or thinks he can stop drinking.

If there is a willingness to try (many times there is), the adolescent should be warned that stopping may cause distress. The family should establish specific guidelines for drug or alcohol use, such as either enter a treatment program or

TABLE 22.1. *Continued.*

		Yes	No
22.	Have you ever been seen at a psychiatric or mental health clinic or gone to any doctor, social worker, or clergyman for help with any emotional problem where drinking was part of the problem?	2	
23.	Have you ever been arrested for drunk driving, driving while intoxicated, or driving under the influence of alcoholic beverages? (If yes, how many times? ____)	2[b]	
24.	Have you ever been arrested or taken into custody, even for a few hours, because of other drunk behavior? (If yes, how many times ____)	2[b]	
25.	Have you ever consciously stopped drinking for a period of time?	2	
26.	Did either of your parents ever have a problem with drinking, or were you ever concerned about either of their drinking?	2	
27.	Have you ever been stopped while driving or apprehended by a law officer for any reason while you were drinking, yet you did not get arrested or receive a citation but probably should have?	2	
28.	Have you ever gone to a doctor for a medical problem, other than liver disease or cirrhosis, that you or he suspected was caused by drinking?	2	
29.	Have you ever been dependent upon or ever had recurring problems with using a drug other than alcohol?	2	

[a] 5 points if delirium tremens.
[b] 2 points for each arrest.

Scoring system:
0–3 Probably not alcoholic
4–5 Borderline
6–7 Possible alcoholic
8–9 80% diagnostic of alcoholism
10+ 100% diagnostic of alcoholism

Adolescents may be slightly overdiagnosed as alcoholics by this screening tool. Some practitioners have adopted a slightly higher score of 13+ as diagnostic of alcoholism. A score of at least 10 indicates a harmful involvement with alcohol, and abstinence should be recommended.

From Davis J, February 1984 (unpublished) and Knox, WJ Objective psychological measurement and alcoholism: Review of the literature, 1971–72. Psychol Rep 38:1023–50, 1976 (Monograph Suppl. 1-V38).

leave the house.[11] Often failure at an attempt to stop drinking is a revelation. Even if there is still much denial and misconception after trying to stop, the patient is more likely to see drinking as a problem and participate in treatment.[9]

Referral and Treatment

For physicians who choose not to manage the demanding complexities of teenage alcoholism themselves, referral presents two dilemmas: the absence of available treatment facilities for adolescents and the difficulty in orchestrating a referral even when there are resources.

A physician can locate what resources are available in the community by a few telephone calls[5]:

1. The State Division of Alcoholism (Ask about services for young people)
2. Alcoholism treatment programs in the community

3. Local child guidance clinic (Ask about staff who work with alcohol- and drug-abusing children)
4. Alcoholics Anonymous (Ask how to find a young people's meeting and then go to it as an observer)
5. Colleagues who treat alcoholics (Ask about resources; physicians who are recovered alcoholics are often especially helpful)
6. Resources from other patients in the physician's own practice (Put a memo on the bulletin board in the waiting room)

Treatment

Teenagers do recover with treatment. In a three-year follow-up study of the Navy's Alcoholism Program, 50% of the patients aged 25 and under had successful outcomes. Older patients had higher success rates.[11]

It is only within the past decade that services that specialize in treatment for adolescent alcoholics have developed. Such services are often expensive and include an inpatient program for a period that ranges from weeks to months. This includes assessment, referral for special problems (such as associated psychiatric illness), contingency contracting, family therapy and education, group therapy with other adolescent alcohol and drug abusers, role playing, and psychodrama. Many experts recommend that an inpatient program be followed by long-term outpatient treatment that includes the adolescent and family for at least three years.[7] While this may seem like a large investment, the cost of undiagnosed and untreated teenage alcoholism in terms of personal and family suffering, public health problems, and economic losses is enormous.

Talking to patients about drinking upsets and embarrasses them, so the impulse is to avoid the confrontation as Mary's doctors did. This reaction is understandable but destructive. A tactful but persistent physician is in a position to accomplish a great deal by making the diagnosis and recommending treatment.

References

1. Department of Health and Human Services: *Fourth Special Report to the US Congress on Alcohol and Health*. 1981:81–1080.
2. Rachal JV, Maisto SA, Guess LL, Hubbard RL: Alcohol use among adolescents, in *Alcohol Consumption and Related Problems*. Alcohol and Health Monograph No 1. Rockville, Md, National Institute of Alcohol Abuse and Alcoholism, 1981.
3. Whitehead P, Ferrence RG: Women and children last: Implications of trends in consumption for women and young people, in Greenblatt M, Schuckit M (eds): *Alcoholism Problems in Women and Children*. New York, Grune & Stratton, 1976.
4. JSL Reports: Alcoholism report. Oct 14, 1982;1–2.
5. Bean M: Identifying and managing alcohol problems in adolescents. *Psychosomatics* 1982;23(4):389–396.

6. Hawthorne W, Menzel N: Youth treatment should be a programming priority. *Alcohol Health Res World* 1983;7(4):46–50.
7. Davis J: Treating the difficult adolescent patient. Presented at American Medical Society on Alcoholism meeting, April 19, 1984. Washington, DC.
8. Donovan J, Jessor R, Jessor L: Problem drinking in adolescence and young adulthood: A follow-up study. *J Stud Alcohol* 1983;44(1):109–137.
9. MeeLee D, Glover LV: The multiproblem addiction patient: Inpatient treatment issues. 1982 (unpublished).
10. Mayer J, Filstead W: The adolescent alcohol involvement scale. *J Stud Alcohol* 1979;40:291–300.
11. Brownell SM: The Navy alcoholism prevention program—worldwide. *Alcoholism Clin Exp Res* 1978;2(4):362–365.

23
The Impaired Physician

W. ANDERSON SPICKARD, JR.

"It is a physician's ethical responsibility to take cognizance of a colleague's inability to practice medicine adequately by reason of physical or mental illness including alcoholism and drug dependence." In 1972, this statement from the *Report of the Council of Mental Health* of the American Medical Association (AMA) emphasized that a national effort was necessary (1) to help impaired physicians return to optimal professional functioning and (2) to safeguard the health of patients from the care rendered by these impaired physicians. Subsequently, medical societies of all 50 states developed procedures to identify and bring into treatment those physicians who were alcohol and drug dependent.[1] Thirty-five states have enacted laws to amend legislation concerned with the practice of medicine so that treatment alternatives are available for impaired physicians involved in disciplinary proceedings.

The AMA now offers a periodic national conference concerned with the problem of the impaired physician, providing an opportunity for members to share ideas and experiences regarding their programs. Although each society has its own unique features, the basic program includes initial identification, intervention, inducement into treatment, rehabilitation, reentry, reeducation, and financial assistance if needed.

The experiences of such centers as the Ridgeview Institute,[2] Mayo Clinic,[3] Menninger Clinic,[4] and the Homewood Sanitarium[5] suggest that treatment for a physician who is alcohol or drug dependent differs from that for nonphysicians.

Prevalence

Because the use of alcohol in combination with other drugs is common in impaired physicians, the incidence of pure alcoholism or pure drug abuse is not known. Despite this classification problem, the incidence of alcoholism and drug problems among physicians is similar to the general population of comparable age, sex, and socioeconomic status.[6] Recent increases in recreational drug use, particularly among medical students and young physicians, reflect societal trends.[7] Six to ten percent of all physicians (22,000 to 36,600) have been, are, or will become alcoholic at some time during their careers.[8,9] Using the Self-Administered Alcoholism Screening Test (SAAST), Niven et al studied the prevalence of alcoholism in a group of 100 physicians attending an annual meeting. He found that 5% were alcoholic and the possibility existed in an additional 2%.[10]

Chemicals Used by Physicians

The Ridgeview Institute conducted the most extensive study of chemically dependent physicians.[2] Gallegos and Norton reviewed the treatment of 675 physicians (650 males and 25 females). Their ethnic background was 96.1% white, 2.4% black, and 1.5% "other." The drugs most frequently abused were alcohol (64.5%), meperidine (30.8%), diazepam (16.5%), amphetamines (12.4%), and pentazocine (10.2%). Most striking was the finding that only 27.2% abused one drug alone, 45.8% abused two to four drugs, 20% five to seven drugs, and 4.7% over seven drugs. One half (52%) took drugs orally only; the rest took drugs orally, intravenously, or intramuscularly. Although no consistent pattern of alcohol and drug abuse was evident among various specialties in the study at Ridgeview, anesthesiologists and physicians in family medicine and emergency medicine seemed to be the most vulnerable.

Progression of Addiction in Alcoholic Physicians

Certain markers in the behavior of physicians suggest that characteristics evident in medical school or earlier may precede alcoholism. An unstable childhood or adolescence,[5,8] unusually perfectionistic behavior, and high academic rank in the graduating class[9] are significant. Drinking patterns during medical school and residency training may correlate with later abuse. Drinking while studying, frequent intoxication, drinking alone, passing out while drinking, and using alcohol to relieve tension and to cope with problems are predictive for subsequent difficulties.

The median age for the first symptoms of addiction is in the mid-40's, after the physician has been in practice for 18 years. The progression of illness in all impaired physicians is remarkably similar. Typically, a physician's practice begins with few patients and responsibilities. In a short time, the practice grows, and family and community responsibilities increase. As the desire for prestige and power increases, the physician assumes he is indispensible and has few limitations.[5] There is excessive concern for detail and reluctance to delegate responsibility. The practice continues to enlarge, the physician becomes too busy, and there is a gradual decrease in outside interests, exercise, family vacations, and spiritual values. Alcohol is used to medicate the stress of overwork and frustration. Fatigue and self-doubts quickly follow, requiring alcohol or drugs to relax and maintain stimulation. Symptoms of allergy, indigestion, bronchitis, fatigue, and insomnia are often the complaints alcoholic physicians use to mask their true illness. When assessed by their colleagues, the true diagnosis of alcoholism is missed. Indecision and depression are severe. Marital discord erupts, and a paramour may be sought. Guilt, depression, and denial become overwhelming, and alcohol or drugs are used in increasing quantity. Psychosis, hopelessness, and even suicide are the end result.

A colleague experienced in the cover-up tactics used by alcoholic physicians must initiate confrontation early in the progression to prevent the usually tragic outcome. A common feature in most alcoholic physicians is tenacious denial. Being a physician and having knowledge of the effects of drugs and alcohol create the delusion that this special insight guarantees immunity. Blindness to the damaging consequences for oneself, family, and patients is aggravated by the lack of acceptance that alcohol dependency is a disease.[11,12] Alcoholic physicians cannot see themselves as sick. Family members and colleagues contribute to the denial by not demanding that the alcoholic seek professional help.

The progressive deterioration of professional skills, family relations, and physical health in the practicing physician is also observed in members of medical school faculties. Colleagues and faculty supervisors deny that the impaired physician is ill and engage in what may be termed the "conspiracy of silence."[13] Confrontation with a colleague's aberrant behavior is delayed for many reasons. First, the use of alcohol is not only condoned but encouraged as consistent with social occasions in medical school faculty events. Second, normal drinking colleagues have experienced the effects of overindulgence and are, therefore, tolerant of those in the early (or even late) stages of alcoholism. Third, repeated drunkenness may be viewed as a response to stress and strain, a form of relaxation under pressure, or merely moral weakness.

The impaired physician on a medical school faculty reacts just as the practicing physician. Behavior leads to a deterioration in job performance. However, the alcoholic faculty member exists in an environment of low supervision, low visibility, freedom from time demands, and vaguely defined standards of performance.[14] Unless supervisors act, the disease often progresses to complete deterioration.

Rehabilitation of the Alcoholic Physician

The alcoholic or drug-addicted, impaired physician is caught in a web of pervasive anxiety, work obsession, and an inexpressible sense of dread.[15] Colleagues and family members must act quickly to stop the downward spiral and induce the physician-patient into treatment.

The process of convincing the physician-patient to undergo treatment is complicated and often frustrating. Concern expressed by a colleague about changes in behavior or performance (without making accusations) is not harmful and, in fact, may be helpful in breaking through denial and starting the patient toward treatment. However, denial may be so intense that all attempts to make the physician-patient aware of improper performance of duties fail. When this occurs, those professionals trained in the process of an intervention should be consulted for assistance. The group trained for this process is the state's Impaired Physician Committee of the Medical Society. Committee members are expert in the process of inducing the alcoholic into treatment and frequently include those recovered from alcoholism or drug addiction. State Impaired Physician Committees are advocacy groups for the impaired physician, emphasizing identification and rehabilitation. If a colleague is willing to go into treatment, a variety of rehabilitation centers is available.

Each state medical society maintains a confidential telephone number to be used by individuals concerned about a colleague suspected of alcoholism. There are two subcommittees in each Impaired Physician Committee: a Verification Subcommittee and a Confrontation Subcommittee. The Verification Subcommittee investigates the report of a person ill with alcoholism and establishes the presence or absence of addiction. Once verified, an organized confrontation is arranged, using members of the Confrontation Subcommittee. The critical step is to get the person into a treatment program, usually an inpatient program followed by a lifelong commitment to aftercare. Despite the emotional trauma of the confrontation, the expense of treatment, and the chance of relapse, a high percentage of physicians treated return to their former positions in practice or on medical school faculties.

The colleague who reports the impaired physician is not guaranteed legal immunity. However, the confidential telephone number at the state medical society is available to protect the anonymity of the caller. Since the initiation of the Impaired Physician's Program in Tennessee, no one has been involved in legal action for reporting an impaired physician.

The first step by the committee of concerned persons is to confront the patient with an accurate history of the alcohol-related behavior, using an attitude of sympathy, compassion, and firmness. At the same time, it is imperative to have strong sanctions in place.[14] After obtaining the full cooperation of family members, care should be taken to coordinate the intervention with partners, employers, or administrative authorities. Coercive methods that may be used are loss of practice privileges in a group practice, suspension of hospital privileges, loss of medical license, or loss of a faculty position.

In rare situations, the confrontation may not be necessary if the impaired physician readily admits to chemical dependency. Usually, however, this is not the case, and the confrontation serves as a vital part of the inducement to treatment. It should usually be carried out by two physicians trained in dealing with denial, anger, and hostility. If members of the family choose to participate, they should be rehearsed so the presentation of facts can be as straightforward, calm, loving, and unemotional as possible.[16] It is important not to make empty threats. Should the physician refuse treatment, the sanctions must be explained carefully and then followed.

In most cases, treatment should take place in an inpatient facility, followed by close observation after discharge. Most rehabilitation programs follow a multidisciplinary approach, which includes peer group therapy, lectures, family therapy, spiritual counseling, exercise, improved nutritional habits, and lessons to refine nonchemical coping skills. Mandated urine checks for drug-addicted physicians increase compliance with the recovery program. Also central to recovery in many instances is attendance at meetings of Alcoholics Anonymous (AA) or Narcotics Anonymous (NA). In many places, there are AA and NA groups just for physicians. After one to two years of intensive treatment, 65% to 75% of physicians are free of alcohol and other drugs.[2,17]

Relapse does occur in some and retreatment is necessary. In a study of 675 physicians, Talbott and Martin[12] identified nine factors that contribute to relapse: (1) lack of acceptance of chemical dependence as a disease, (2) continued denial, (3) pressure of a dysfunctional family system, (4) dishonesty, (5) lack of a spiritual program, (6) cross-addiction, (7) stress, (8) emotional or physical traps of hunger, loneliness, fatigue, self-pity, and (9) isolation. Relapse usually occurred within one or two years of treatment, and failure to recognize the warning signs led to tragic consequences.

For the recovered alcoholic physician, reentry into practice or return to a faculty position after treatment is difficult. Feelings of guilt, inadequacy, and the craving for alcohol or drugs do not disappear quickly or easily after treatment. If the alcoholic physician follows the prescribed recovery program, successful, lifelong rehabilitation results. Successful recovery is enhanced by sympathetic encouragement and support from colleagues, family, and friends.

References

1. Steindler EM: Physician impairment: Past, present, future. *J Med Assoc G* 1984; 73:741–743.
2. Gallegos KV, Norton M: Characterization of Georgia's impaired physicians program treatment population: Data and statistics. *J Med Assoc G* 1984;73:755–758.
3. Morse RM, Martin MA, Swenson WM, Niven RG: Prognosis of physicians treated for alcoholism and drug dependence. *JAMA* 1984;251:743–746.
4. Johnson RP, Connelly JC: Addicted physicians: A closer look. *JAMA* 1981;245:253–257.
5. Vincent MO, Robinson EA, Latt L: Physicians as patients: Private psychiatric hospital experience. *Can Med Assoc J* 1969;100:403–412.
6. Brewster JM: Prevalence of alcoholism and other drug problems among physicians. *JAMA* 1986;55:1913–1920.
7. McAuliffe WE, Rohman M, Santangelo S, et al: Psychoactive drug use among practicing physicians and medical students. *N Engl J Med* 1986;315:805–810.
8. Vaillant GE, Sobowale NC, McArthur C: Some psychologic vulnerabilities of physicians. *N Engl J Med* 1972;287:372–375.
9. Bissell L, Jones RW: The alcoholic physician: A survey. *Am J Psychiatry* 1976;133:1142–1146.
10. Niven RG, Hurt RD, Morse RM, Swenson WM: Alcoholism in physicians. *Mayo Clin Proc* 1984;59:12–16.
11. Butcher TE, Talbott GD: Dynamics in group process in impaired health professionals. *J Med Assoc G* 1984;771–774.

12. Talbott GD, Martin CA: Relapse and recovery: Special issues for chemically dependent physicians. *J Med Assoc G* 1984;73:763–769.
13. Spickard A Jr, Billings FT: Alcoholism in a medical school faculty. *N Engl J Med* 1981;305:1646–1648.
14. Thoreson RW: The professor at risk: Alcohol abuse in academe, in Thoreson, RW, Hosokawa EP (eds): *Employee Assistance Programs in Higher Education*. Springfield, Ill, Charles C Thomas, 1984, pp 123–143.
15. Thoreson RW: The professional executive alcoholic: Sabbatical perspective. *Almacan* 1981;11:5.
16. Spickard A, Thompson BR: *Dying for a Drink– What You Should Know About Alcoholism*. Waco, Tex, Word Publishers, Inc., 1985, pp 102–136.
17. Shore JH: The impaired physician: Four years after probation. *JAMA* 1982;248:3127–3130.

24 The Patient with Mixed-Substance Abuse

ROGELIO D. BAYOG

Alcohol abuse, combined with abuse of other substances, is a growing public health problem. People referred to a physician for drug-related problems are likely to report use of more than one type of psychoactive drug. A large-scale longitudinal study by Craddock et al of more than 11,000 clients seen in a drug treatment center from 1979 to 1981[1] indicated that drug users who entered treatment during this period had complex drug and alcohol use patterns. A typical client used alcohol, marijuana, and heroin several times a week plus cocaine several times a month (as well as other narcotics and minor tranquilizers at least monthly). Although there is a first drug of choice, many patients commonly use other mood-altering substances to treat withdrawal, modify the experience of intoxication, or change the high.

Multiple drug use often starts in adolescence. Nearly two thirds of American young people will try an illicit drug before they finish high school.[2] About one student in 20 is using marijuana and/or alcohol on a daily basis, and 40% of students surveyed report having five or more drinks consecutively on at least one occasion in the prior two weeks.[2] These figures add up to an impressive 3.5 million adolescents between the ages of 14 and 17 who have abnormal patterns of drinking. In contrast, nicotine is less popular as a drug of choice, with 29% of adolescents reporting smoking in the past month.

Types of Addictive Drugs

Commonly abused drugs can be classified according to their pharmacologic action, their psychoactive effects, or their potential for causing addiction. One such classification includes stimulants, depressants, hallucinogens, inhalants, and marijuana. The distinction between drugs that cause dependence versus abuse is often misleading because the potential for addiction does not correlate with the severity of the problems from drug use. For instance, consumption of caffeine, which produces symptoms of tolerance and withdrawal (pathognomonic for an addicting drug), is not associated with the morbidity and mortality seen with abuse of cocaine, which does not cause the same type of physiologic addiction. The powerful euphoriant effect of cocaine and postcocaine dysphoria strongly reinforce compulsive drug use, which rapidly leads to loss of choice and loss of control over drug use. Craving for short-lived cocaine euphoria is so compelling that many cocaine users spend all their time, energy, and money to procure and use cocaine to the exclusion of everything else. Behaviorally, there is clear bondage to the drug, even though classic withdrawal has not been described.

Nicotine is another drug that confounds the usual classifications. The dangers of smoking tobacco are not the result of addiction to the stimulant nicotine but, rather, to the long-term deleterious effects of smoking on the cardiovascular and respiratory systems. However, the addictive properties of nicotine perpetuate widespread use of cigarettes despite known adverse consequences and lead to a high relapse among those smokers who try to quit.

The terminology for mixed-substance abuse is often confusing. In *Diagnostic and Statistical Manual of Mental Disorders-III*,[3] mixed substance abuse or dependence is diagnosed when substances abused are from more than one nonalcoholic substance category, for example, amphetamines and barbiturates. A distinction of dubious clinical usefulness is made between polydrug and multidrug use. Polydrug abuse reflects use of more than one psychoactive substance, except opiates. Multidrug abuse includes those who use two psychoactive substances other than alcohol, nicotine, caffeine, or prescribed medications. As the epidemiology suggests, the combination of drugs used is often too full to list, and the clinician often prefers not to identify the drugs singly.

Initial Assessment

When a patient comes to the physician with a drug problem, it is important to take a careful history, perform a thorough physical examination, and obtain basic laboratory data. Addicts are generally poor historians, making it particularly useful to have a collateral source of information, for example, a spouse, parent, or significant other.

In the course of gathering data for differential diagnosis, the following questions should be answered to formulate a treatment strategy:

1. What is the problem that brings the patient to treatment?
2. How severe is the addiction?
3. Is the mixed-substance abuse a primary problem, or is it secondary to underlying mental illness, such as schizophrenia, depression, antisocial personality, or atypical psychosis?
4. What is the primary drug problem, and what is the extent of use?
5. Can the patient be treated on an outpatient basis, or should he be admitted to the hospital?

The Presenting Problem

A life-threatening situation, such as drug intoxication or withdrawal, pressure from spouse, employer, or legal system, a concurrent or complicating medical illness, are common reasons why patients seek help. Their problems, whether antecedent to or the result of addiction, are often complex and frustrating and tax the patience and tolerance of the clinician. In looking for help for their addiction, addicts may state a different chief complaint.

LR, a 36-year-old divorced Hispanic male, comes to the emergency unit of a Veterans Administration Hospital complaining of depression with suicidal ideation. Preliminary assessment reveals important losses, ie, breaking up with his girlfriend and recently losing his job. Although he initially denies having a drug problem, he later states that he has abused multiple drugs, including heroin daily, cocaine 1 g three to four times a week, and alcohol two to five drinks daily. He is desperate and physically sick. Afraid he will not get admitted, he emphasizes suicidality.

He was treated for drug withdrawal and then referred to the therapeutic community program which he completed. Follow-up found him drug free after one year.

The Severity of the Addiction

The existence of psychologic, legal, employment, medical, and social problems related to drug use are sensitive indicators of the seriousness of the addiction and identify complications that must be addressed.

The Primary Problem

Understanding whether a mixed-substance abuse problem is primary or secondary is not as important initially as knowing what conditions need immediate treatment. Clearly emergency conditions due to intoxication or withdrawal or the possibility of danger to self or others are managed first to keep the patient safe. Subsequently, a patient with a mixed-substance abuse problem can be evaluated for major psychiatric illness. Because symptoms of substance abuse, such as confusion, delusions, hallucinations, impaired memory, and poor judgment,[4,5] can mimic most major psychiatric problems, a final diagnosis may require several weeks of observation.

The Primary Drug of Abuse

The extent of drug use is of little value in determining prognosis. However, identification of the primary drug of abuse has therapeutic implications. Patients who abuse narcotics suffer primarily from the disorganizing and threatening effects of rage and aggression.[6–8] Those who abuse cocaine and other stimulants self-medicate underlying depression and its equivalents. Since many addicts cannot identify or describe how they feel, this information may help the clinician interpret the patient's distress and provide appropriate help.

Type of Treatment

In principle, drug addicts should be treated on an outpatient basis whenever possible. Outpatient programs are cheaper, less regressive, and cause less disruption in their family and work life, the latter being important if the addict is the sole source of family support. Patients who do well in outpatient treatment are motivated for recovery, have a supportive social network, can keep their counseling appointments regularly (with or without the family), participate in a urine screening program or other contingencies, that is, sign a contract to allow the clinic to inform their employer or parole officer if they show drugs in the urine or report intoxicated, and have an affinity for self-help groups.

The following is a partial list of indications for inpatient treatment:

1. Medical complications of drug use, such as subacute bacterial endocarditis, fulminant hepatitis, septicemia
2. Life-threatening intoxication or withdrawal syndromes, such as seizures, coma
3. Need to stop a cycle of drug taking that is out of control
4. Psychiatric emergencies, such as major depression with high risk of suicide, combative behavior, toxic psychosis
5. Patients with no money, no home, no job
6. Those mandated by the courts to attend a treatment program in lieu of jail (Surprisingly, addicts in enforced treatment do well. In one report, 95% completed residential treatment and returned for outpatient follow-up for one year[9])
7. Those whose psychosocial status reinforces continuing drug use in spite of repeated attempts to stop through self-help groups, clinics, or private therapists

Treatment

Once the assessment is complete, the physician should formulate a concrete treatment plan and discuss it with the patient and family. Meyer has described the four kinds of services required in the rehabilitation of addicts: (1) treatment of overdosage, (2) treatment of the withdrawal syndrome, (3) treatment of medical and psychosocial complications, and (4) modification of chronic relapsing behaviors.[10] This framework clarifies the goals of the therapist and provides a guide for the patient and the clinician during the course of treatment. The physician can decide to be involved with some or all of these services. Regardless of the degree of involvement, the physician should understand several principles of treatment.

Developing a Therapeutic Relationship

The physician should take the opportunity in any phase of treatment to develop a good patient-physician relationship. This is based on trust and rapport engendered by the doctor's genuine interest, respect, and empathy for the patient, as well as the patient's motivation to be helped. The offer of help instills hope, with resulting relief of anxiety.

This relationship can be threatened at the onset if the physician does not understand the way the addict behaves. The patient's behavior when intoxicated or in withdrawal represents regression to a lower level of functioning mediated through changes in the CNS. This type of behavior can be infantile, demanding, impulsive, aggressive, or passive and withdrawn. It can elicit anxiety, fear, rage, frustration, and even contempt and guilt from the caregiver. It is easy to abandon a caring and hopeful posture when both the doctor and patient need it most. The biggest challenge is to engage the patient in treatment so that the addict realizes that the therapeutic relationship with the physician or counselor can eventually be a viable substitute for drugs. This is possible when the doctor genuinely cares for, respects, and even loves the patient and views him as a unique, susceptible individual with specific strengths and weaknesses who now suffers from a serious behavioral disorder and needs help.

Patient and Physician Attitudes

Physician and patient attitudes are important in the beginning to establish what could be, at best, a fragile alliance. The reactions these patients elicit from their doctors and other caregivers have to be understood. Doctors become symbols of significant figures in the patient's early life. If the parents were cruel, domineering, inconsistent, incompetent, or depriving, the patient reacts as though the physician is the same or, alternatively, pushes the physician to be punitive and withholding. Clearly, this is an unconscious or conditionally learned level of functioning. Given this insight, it is important not to punish or reject addicts even when they literally ask for it. Rather, knowledge of the details that brought the patient to the treatment situation can help deepen the therapeutic relationship. This knowledge can also be used to set realistic limits, confront, and offer an emotional climate that helps the addict contain feelings of rage, shame, anxiety, loneliness, and poor self-esteem.

In spite of the clinician's best efforts, patients will sometimes defeat clinical approaches. They flee from treatment or return to drug use. Relapse has many meanings, including the need for relief, a conditioned response, or a defiant or aggressive act. Sometimes relapse can represent a positive response to treatment. The addict may need to test a new understanding of his drug problem by experimenting with drugs again. Similarly, the anxiety engendered in a successful effort to make significant lifestyle and personality changes may result in occasional relapses. At this point, the physician's reserves of tolerance, patience, and optimism will be taxed to the limit in containing the impulse to retaliate and discontinue treatment.

The physician should always keep in mind that, although some patients stop or cut down drug use after their first attempt at treatment, substance abuse is a chronic disease with frequent exacerbations and remissions.

Individualize the Treatment Plan

No two addicts are alike. A good initial assessment makes this clear to the physician. Treatment must be directed toward the individual's needs. Areas such as interpersonal relationships, physical health, vocational status, and psychologic health are considered in the assessment, treatment, and outcome.

Use of Medications

The substitution of drugs to treat addiction and deal with underlying conflict and problems should be avoided whenever possible. Neuroleptic drugs are indicated for psychotic episodes in patients with schizophrenia, major affective disorders, and transient severe reactions. Antidepressants may be used for major depression and some phobic disorders, to lower craving for cocaine, or to decrease the severity of withdrawal syndromes from stimulant drugs. Sedative-hypnotic and anxiolytic drugs are of little or no value except on a strict, time-limited basis to establish diurnal rhythm and for adjustment disorders. Their capacity to produce craving due to cross-tolerance contraindicates their use further in many patients.

Treatment of Overdosage and Withdrawal Syndromes

This is beyond the scope of this book, and readers are referred to several excellent summaries.[11,12]

Rehabilitation

Since polydrug abuse is a chronic behavioral disorder, treatment does not stop in the acute phase. The initial goal of rehabilitation is to stop drug use. Patients experience remarkable improvement in cognitive functioning and judgment when they first become abstinent. This permits intervention in physical and psychosocial problems that need immediate attention. Bean-Bayog[13] lists several steps required of the patient in order to recover from addiction:

1. Enter drug treatment program and establish a therapeutic alliance.
2. Learn the reasons to stay abstinent—essentially, that the use of a single or several doses of the drug is likely to cause slow or rapid readdiction and suffering.
3. Learn how to stay abstinent with the use of self-help groups, counseling, clinics, or by substituting people for drugs.
4. Cope with the consequences of stopping drug use: painful feelings, finding other avenues of relief, added responsibility and demands, all leading to vulnerability for relapse.
5. Grieve the losses secondary to addiction, such as a spouse, children, prestige, money, and lost experiences.
6. Obtain psychiatric treatment for underlying or complicating emotional illness. Neuroleptics for thought disorder or psychotherapy for anxiety and depression may be needed.

Although the primary care physician may decide not to undertake the labor-intensive work of rehabilitation, it is important to be familiar with treatment approaches and treatment systems so that the patient can be referred properly.

Treatment Approaches and Treatment Systems

Costello's review of treatment systems for alcoholics is also applicable to patients with mixed-substance abuse.[14] The programs have the following characteristics: (1) a well-organized treatment philosophy implemented in a consistent and logical fashion, (2) inpatient resources for medical care and nonmedical rehabilitation, (3) aggressive outreach linkage with community agencies, both to bring patients to attention through community contacts and to effect transition back into the community, and (4) behaviorally oriented interventions, in addition to strictly verbal therapies.

Most therapies used to treat alcoholics are also used in the treatment of mixed-substance abuse. Individual therapy ranges from insight-oriented psychotherapy (not indicated routinely) to various behavioral programs (reviewed by Stitzer et al).[15] Family therapy can be very helpful in situations where the sick role of the addict is used by the family to maintain its own homeostasis. Residential programs focus either on maintaining a safe, drug-free environment while the addict reintegrates himself into society (halfway houses) or on helping the addict make more substantial personality changes through intensive group therapy experience (therapeutic community programs).

One treatment program that explicitly uses drugs in therapy is the methadone maintenance program. Methadone was introduced in the United States by Dole and Nyswander.[17] It is an effective approach in preventing illicit opioid use among narcotic addicts. Though some patients continue to dabble in mixed-drug use, this practice is reduced. Among patients actively involved in these programs, there is a decrease in drug-related crimes and better involvement with their families. More time is spent at work and less time in jail.

Self-help groups, such as Cocaine Anonymous and Narcotics Anonymous, instill hope and provide a place for acceptance and social networking. They create opportunities to share the pains of addiction and the joys of recovery, and to learn about the resiliency of people. Patterned after AA, they emphasize spirituality, making amends to people injured by the addict, correcting one's character flaws, and helping other addicts to enhance one's own recovery process. The only requirement is that the patient wants to stop using drugs. It is not a requirement to admit that one is an addict. These groups are rapidly growing in acceptance and participation.

Prognosis

The efficacy of treatment in mixed-substance abuse varies according to several factors.[1] General statements can be made about outcomes:

1. Treated addicts do better than those not treated at all.
2. Patients who are socioeconomically advantaged, have jobs, and are highly motivated do well.
3. Older clients with prior treatment experiences show less alcohol use, more drug-related problems, less criminal behavior, less depression, and less drug usage while in treatment.
4. Patients who abuse multiple drugs (excluding opiates) have less positive outcomes during treatment.
5. Although patients may continue illicit drug use during drug treatment, they do significantly less compared to pretreatment data. Substituting one drug for another is common (eg, alcohol for opiates).
6. Dropout rates are higher in drug-free treatment programs (whether residential or outpatient).
7. The mortality rate is not accurately known but is high.
8. Patients who drop out often return to some form of treatment selected on the basis of their usage pattern.
9. Adequate data are not available about patients who abuse mixed drugs and recover without treatment.

References

1. Craddock SG, Brady RM, Hubbard RL: *Drug Use Before and During Drug Abuse Treatment:* 1979–1981, TOPS admission cohorts. (DHHS Publication No (ADM) 85–1387), 1985:13–30.
2. Johnston LD, O'Malley PM, Bachman JG: *Use of Licit and Illicit Drugs by America's High School Students*, 1975–1984. (DHHS Publication No (ADM) 85–1394), 1985:9–15.
3. American Psychiatric Association: *Diagnostic and Statistical Manual of Mental Disorders-III*. Washington, DC, APA, 1980, pp 163–179.
4. Schuckit MA: Alcoholism and affective disorder: Diagnostic confusion, in Goodwin DW, Erickson CK (eds): *Alcoholism and Affective Disorders*. New York, SP Medical & Scientific Books, 1979.
5. Goodwin DW, Alderson P, Rosenthal R: Clinical significance of hallucinations in psychiatric disorders. *Arch Gen Psychiatry* 1971;24:76–80.
6. Krystal H, Raskin HA: *Drug Dependence: Aspects of Ego Functions*. Detroit, Wayne State University Press, 1970.
7. Wurmser L: Psychoanalytic considerations of the etiology of compulsive drug use. *J Am Psychoanalyt Assoc* 1974;22:820–843.
8. Khantzian EJ: The self-medication hypothesis of addictive disorders: Focus on heroin and cocaine dependence. *Am J Psychiatry* 1985;142:1259–1264.
9. Deneault P, Correira R, Taviera A, Andrews R: Outcome study in a therapeutic community program for polydrug abusers. Unpublished report, 1980.
10. Meyer RE: *Guide to Drug Rehabilitation, A Public Health Response*. Boston: Beacon Press, 1972.
11. Schuckit MA: *Drug and Alcohol Abuse*. New York, Plenum Press, 1984.
12. Dykens JW, Bayog RD: The treatment of drug addiction, in Wolman BB (ed): *The Therapist's Handbook*. New York, Van Nostrand Rheinhold Company, 1983, pp 483–505.

13. Bean-Bayog M: Alcoholism treatment as an alternative to psychiatric hospitalization. *Psychiat Clin North Am* 1985;8(3):501–512.
14. Costello RM: Alcoholism treatment and evaluation. I. In search of methods. *Int J Addictions* 1975;10:251–275.
15. Stitzer ML, Bigelow GE, McCaul ME: *Behavior Therapy in Drug Abuse Treatment: Review and Evaluation*. DHHS Publication No (ADM) 85–1401, 1985:31–50.
16. Bayog RD, Fisch A: Family evaluation in a methadone maintenance clinic. *Trans Mental Health Res* 1979;21:28–32.
17. Dole VP, Nyswander M: Medical treatment of heroin addiction. *JAMA* 1965;193(8):646–650.
18. National Institute of Drug Abuse and National Institute on Alcohol Abuse and Alcoholism: *National Directory of Drug Abuse and Alcoholism and Prevention Programs*. (DHHS Publication No (ADM) 85–321), 1985.

Part VII
Ethical and Legal Issues

Introduction to Ethical and Legal Issues in the Treatment of Alcoholism

Grodin, Hingson, and Meyers bring the practitioner up to date on the legal and ethical implications of treating the alcoholic patient. Using the paradigm of drunk driving as the focal point, they discuss differences between the ethical and legal responsibilities borne by the primary physician, the emergency room physician, the physician working for law enforcement agencies, and the court physician. They sketch the rights of patients, demonstrating how physicians may inadvertently, yet illegally, invade their privacy. They discuss under what circumstances blood should be drawn to evaluate for drug dependency and emphasize the proper role of record keeping.

25 Ethical and Legal Issues in the Treatment of Alcoholism: Drunk Driving

MICHAEL GRODIN, RALPH HINGSON, and ALLAN MEYERS

The role and responsibility of the practicing physician with respect to patients with alcoholism is fraught with medical, legal, and philosophical quandaries. When does a physician's concern for the welfare of the patient become paternalistic at the expense of the patient's autonomy? When, if ever, can physicians draw blood-alcohol levels (BALs) on a patient without his consent? Who should have access to patients' records with regard to alcoholism? Does concern for the public's safety ever override the commitment to patient confidentiality? How certain must a physician be of a diagnosis of alcoholism before taking action to protect the patient or the public? What are the limits, implications, and justifications for such actions? Who establishes the rules for the doctor-patient relationship, and what are the goals of that interaction?

These questions establish a groundwork for critical explorations into the appropriate nature of a physician's involvement with alcoholic patients, whether it be as primary physician, agent of social control, society's gatekeeper, or protector of the public health and well-being. The physician's response to and responsibility for drunk drivers brings all these questions into focus.

Ethical and Legal Perspectives on the Patient-Physician Relationship

The nature of the physician-patient relationship has been described metaphorically in terms of contract, covenant, friendship, and acquaintance.[1] The basis of this relationship is mutual trust and respect, with the implicit goal of working together in an attempt to reach the patient's life goals or concept of health and wellness.[2] If this unique relationship is to result in responsible interchange, certain ethical presuppositions must form a framework.[3] The principle of respect for other people demands that physicians promote autonomous decision making in their patients. Practically, this translates morally and legally into the doctrine of informed consent. No autonomous individual should be touched or treated without his informed and explicit consent. A further extension of the notion of respect for persons is that nonautonomous people should not be allowed to make incompetent decisions, as this would be to disrespect them. Decisions affecting such a person should be based either on that person's previously autonomous statements or on an understanding of the patient's value system. Without prior knowledge of the patient's values, decisions should be based on what appears to be that person's best interests. Finally, decisions might be based on what a reasonable person might wish. The emphasis on such decision making appropriately focuses on the individual's autonomous rights and medical welfare as the paramount—if not sole—concern. Justification is required for any actions that might be carried out against a competent patient's will. Such paternalistic actions could be justified only if such beneficient interventions were directed toward the patient's best interests and well-being. Respect for people also requires prima facie respect for patient confidentiality and consistent honesty.

These ethical precepts governing the nature of the doctor-patient relationship can be applied in the case of alcoholism or drunk driving. Physicians must be honest and trustworthy in their discussions with patients and should ensure their patients' autonomous decision making through the doctrine of informed consent. Physicians and patients should expect a relationship of mutual respect. The alcoholic person should be told of his condition and assured the strictest confidentiality. Neither police, insurers, nor any third party should have access to medical records without the patient's consent or without specific laws that require reporting by physicians. No laboratory studies, including BALs, should be performed without the explicit or implicit consent of the autonomous patient, unless laws mandate the physician to act. Although reporting is mandatory for some infectious diseases, in many states there is no law requiring mandatory reporting of drunk drivers. Confidentiality of patients' records in alcoholism or drug treatment programs is mandated by federal statute. Data should be used solely to help benefit the patient in his endeavors toward health and well-being. Patients who are inebriated or who have a decreased level of consciousness should have only those laboratory tests medically indicated to maximize benefit to the patient.

Although patients may disagree with a physician's diagnosis of alcohol or drug dependence and may even request that such diagnoses not be entered in their records, it is a physician's responsibility to enter into the record the most complete and accurate diagnoses he can make. The patient should be told and the reasons for disagreement discussed. However, a diagnosis should be made and subsequently recorded in the patient's medical record only if it has direct significance for patient care, with implications for therapy and prognosis. In discussing the diagnosis with the patient, the physician should be sensitive to the use of value judgments, the medicalization of social and public policy concerns, and the stigma often associated with indiscriminate labeling. Any deviation from these ethical norms not only requires the knowledge of the patient but also must be made explicit, verifiable, and justifiable.

Nature of the Medical Care Setting and Physician-Patient Relationship

A 33-year-old housewife sees her physician frequently for minor physical complaints, most of which are related to her heavy alcohol intake. She relates a history of frequent episodes of driving while intoxicated, including several near-accidents when driving her children home from school.

In this particular state, state law mandates physicians to report cases of possible child abuse or neglect, and the physician must consider whether these episodes warrant further investigation. He begins by sharing with the patient his concerns about the risk to her children of her driving while drunk in an effort to help her obtain appropriate treatment. He also informs her of his obligation to file a report of possible neglect if she is unable to change her behavior.

The physical and administrative setting in which the physician-patient encounter occurs often has significant implications for the rules under which the relationship takes place. In the continuity of a primary care setting, the physician and patient develop a relationship over time. They know each other and are clear on the ground rules. There is little question that the physician is working and advocating for the patient. The ethical norms of autonomy, consent, and confidentiality are upheld, with paternalism reserved for rare and justified situations. In such practice, there should be little confusion with respect to these norms. The primary care provider who gives episodic care or works within a large group will be less likely to know the patient and, thus, may have more difficulty with notions of autonomy and confidentiality. The goals and ground rules, however, remain constant.

A 21-year-old man is brought to the emergency room by police ambulance following a motor vehicle accident. He is conscious but confused. He has sustained lacerations and contusions to his head and has an odor of alcohol on his breath. His uninjured fellow passengers state that they had been to a party where there were alcohol and other drugs available. The police request a report on his medical condition.

In an emergency room setting, the environment, goals, and procedures for dealing with an intoxicated patient may differ. Although the focus should still be on medical indications for evaluation and laboratory testing and treating the patient, other competing values come into play. If the patient is combative, uncooperative, or a danger to himself or others, physicians may be forced to treat without consent and even to draw diagnostic studies to help elucidate the clinical condition. An intoxicated person who refuses treatment and intends to drive away from a hospital emergency room setting should be offered alternate transportation. If the person persists, he should be informed that the medical staff will contact the police because of the threat that person's intoxicated driving could pose to others. The degree to which there is impairment of autonomy or risks to personnel, in conjunction with uncertain historical information, may necessitate a more paternalistic stance. Even in the emergency room, physicians must be clear that the goals of therapy should be medical diagnosis, therapy, and rehabilitation. Yet physicians are not law-enforcement agents, and they cannot, nor should they, test BALs or divulge information about patients who agree to treatment unless there is consent, statutory regulation, or a court order. It is most important that patients realize that physicians are their advocates and will be justified in taking paternalistic actions only if they are carried out on incompetent patients. They must be assured that such interventions would occur only when significant harm could occur without intervention, that the benefits outweigh those harms, and that the intervention is as unintrusive and respectful as possible.

Even if a police officer requests that the emergency room physician draw blood without a specific court order, the physician is under no obligation to do so. That does not mean, however, that the state cannot obtain BALs from patients. Police departments can hire their own physicians. Most states also have implied consent laws, which mean that when drivers obtain their licenses they are giving the police consent to test them for BALs if the police have probable cause to believe the individual was driving while intoxicated (DWI). Probable cause can be provided by such occurrences as the odor of alcohol, presence of alcohol in a vehicle, slurred speech, weaving in traffic, or involvement in a crash. In most states, failure of the driver to submit to a breath or blood test is punishable by fine or license suspension equal to or greater than the penalties for DWI.

Settings that pose a more ambiguous or frankly adversarial posture toward patient care and autonomy also exist. For example, physicians who practice occupational medicine may not always have the patient's rights, autonomy, and confidentiality as a paramount concern. Employers may want access to any information regarding alcoholism in the workplace, instances of DWI, or any substance abuse leading to impairment in an employee's functioning or absenteeism. This is a situation in which the quality of work could affect the safety of others, for example, people who make or operate planes, trucks, or automobiles. The physician in such a setting may serve as the agent of both the patient and the company, and both the patient and the doctor may be employees of the company. Another example is the physician who carries out physical examinations or screenings for insurance companies. What is important for physicians to consider in these instances is that patients should be made aware of potential conflicts of interest, goals, and procedures that comprise the ground rules for that particular setting. In general, patients should understand and consent to the package that may come with such settings. The inherent conflict of interest in such a relationship requires a different form and structure for ethical precepts.

A physician who is in the employ of the police, court, or criminal justice system will not have the patient's or suspect's interest as a priority, and the physician in such a case may actually be the agent of the state. The patient or suspect should be told explicitly about the ground rules under which such a physician is operating, but he may not be given the opportunity to consent to the relationship. Still other considerations may come from public health statutes regarding the reporting of alcoholism and alcohol-related diseases. Criminal laws may require reporting specific alcohol-related activities that are statutory violations or criminal offenses. The public-at-large appears to appreciate these constraints on confidentiality, which are universal to all professional relationships.

A Primary Care Approach to the Drunk Driver

Not all physicians approach the patient who drives while drunk in the same manner. However, as a baseline, a primary physician must understand the scope of the problem of drunk driving, the patients most at risk, and the treatment available to counteract drunk driving behavior. Traffic accidents claimed 44,241 lives in 1984.[4] During the past decade, they were the leading cause of death for people under age 35.[5] The risk of being involved in a traffic crash increases with a BAL of 0.05 g/dL, the equivalent of two to three drinks on an empty stomach.[6] Physicians should query all patients involved in traffic crashes about their drinking. Approximately one third of drivers involved in fatal accidents have BALs exceeding 0.10 g/dL, the legal limit for intoxication in many states.[6] One driver in three involved in a crash resulting in serious injuries had been drinking,[7] and one half of those involved in fatal crashes had consumed at least some alcohol before the crash.

At all ages, men are more likely than women to engage in drunk driving and be involved in crashes. Young men under the age of 25 are at particular risk for fatal motor vehicle accidents.[4-7] Although they represent only 10% of drivers, their lack of driving experience and their propensity for risk-taking behavior in traffic (eg, speeding, running red lights, driving after drinking or using drugs, and not wearing seatbelts) result in their involvement in 26% of fatal accidents.[8] Although drunk driving does not necessarily imply that the patient has alcoholism, known alcoholics are also at increased risk for motor vehicle accidents associated with drinking.[6]

Having identified the high-risk patient, the physician should educate him about the risks associated with his behavior. An opportune time for discussion comes when the patient gives the history of an accident; at that point, the consequences of drunk driving are undeniable. Additional information about how alcohol impairs driving performance may be helpful. Because, as noted above, drunk drivers as a group disproportionately tend to engage in a variety of riskful behaviors while driving, the patient should also be queried and counseled about these other risks.

The physician may care for some patients who are participating in court-ordered treatment programs. Although these programs may help certain individuals, there is little evidence that they reduce drunk driving or alcohol-associated accidents.[10-14] One important reason may be that patients are given treatment involuntarily. A goal for the physician is to encourage patients to seek help voluntarily. The physician may be able to use the patient's reactions to a mandated program to develop a more helpful voluntary treatment program.

Although a physician has a right and even an obligation to speak out in the public forum regarding societal policy and procedures, there must not be any confusion about the first, and sole, obligation: to be an advocate for the patient. Physicians must not intermingle or confuse their roles and must be explicit about when and where such trust could be violated. This ethical imperative is most striking in the dilemma associated with the care of patients who suffer from alcoholism or who are drunk drivers. Physicians have a difficult role to play in the lives of their patients suffering from alcoholism, and they also have an opportunity to address in a significant way the major public health problem of drunk driving. Physicians must recognize the opportunities presented when treating a patient who has been driving drunk. They must use this event as a crucial entry point to address the patient's self-destructive course. Physicians should do this for the patient, for the innocent victims of drunk drivers, and for the public-at-large.

References

1. Childress J: *Who Should Decide? Paternalism in Health Care*. New York, Oxford University Press, 1982.
2. Katz J: *The Silent World of Doctor and Patient*. New York, Free Press, 1984.
3. Beauchamp T, Childress J: *Principles of Biomedical Ethics*. New York, Oxford University Press, 1983.
4. US Department of Transportation: *Fatal Accident Reporting System, 1984*. DOT HS 806 919, 1986.
5. Ross HL: *Deterring the Drinking Driver, Legal Policy and Social Control*. Lexington, Mass, Lexington Books, 1982.
6. *Fifth Special Report to the US Congress on Alcohol and Health. Adverse Social Consequences of Alcohol Use and Alcoholism*. DHHS publication No ADM 84 1291, 1984.
7. US Department of Transportation: *1984: A Report on Traffic Accidents and Injuries in the US*. DOT HS 806 867, 1985.
8. Wagenaar AC, Douglas RL, Compt CP, Pett LC: Raising the legal drinking age in Michigan and Maine. Rockville, Md, Report N2UM HSR1 58-81.
9. Council on Scientific Affairs: Alcohol and the driver. *JAMA* 1986;255:522-527.
10. US Department of Transportation: *Fatal accident reporting system, 1984. A Review of the State of Knowledge*. DOT HS 806 569, 1985, p 13.
11. Levy P, Voas R, Johnson P, Klein JM: An evaluation of the Department of Transportation's alcohol safety action projects. *J Safety Res* 1978;10(4):162-176.
12. Nichols JL, Weinstein EB, Ellinstad VS, Struckman-Johnson DL: The specific deterrent effect of ASAA education and rehabilitation programs. *J Safety Res* 1978; 10(4):177-187.
13. Insurance Institute for Highway Safety Highway Loss Reduction Status Report. 1979;14(6).
14. Reis Jr RE: *The Effects of DUI Education and Counseling Programs on Recidivism*. Prepared for the Workshop on Alcohol and the Drinking Driver. Sponsored by the National Institute on Alcohol Abuse and Alcoholism and the National Highway Traffic Safety Administration. Bethesda, Md, May 2-4, 1984.

Annotated References

General Concepts and Clinical Pharmacology

Bean MH: Denial and the psychological complications of alcoholism, in Bean MH, Zinberg NE (eds): *Dynamic Approaches to the Understanding and Treatment of Alcoholism*. New York, Free Press, 1981, pp 55–96.

Excellent discussion of the clinical manifestations of denial and some therapeutic strategies for helping the denying alcoholic.

Behnke RH: Recognition and management of alcohol withdrawal syndrome. *Hosp Pract* 1976;11:79–84.

A study of the practical aspects of therapy for withdrawal syndrome.

Clark WD: Alcoholism: Blocks to diagnosis and treatment. *Am J Med* 1981; 71:275–286.

A coherent, persuasive defense of the disease concept of alcoholism offering useful advice on diagnosis and treatment.

Edwards G, Gross MM: Alcohol dependence: Provisional description of a clinical syndrome. *Br Med J* 1976;1:1058–1061.

An articulate, brief, seminal article on clinical characteristics of the alcohol dependence syndrome.

Fein R: *Alcohol in America: The Price We Pay.* Newport Beach, Calif, CareInstitute, 1984.

A succinct analysis of the economic impact of alcohol.

Fifth Special Report to the US Congress on Alcohol and Health. Rockville, Md, DHHS Publication No (ADM) 84-1291, 1983.

A rich summary of the epidemiology of alcohol use and abuse.

Hawkins RD, Kalant H: The metabolism of ethanol and its metabolic effects. *Pharmacol Rev* 1972;24:67–157.

The definitive account of ethanol pharmacokinetics and pharmacokinetic interactions with other drugs.

Johnson VE: *I'll Quit Tomorrow.* New York, Harper and Row, 1975.

Major proponent of family-intervention techniques discusses how alcoholism develops and why intervention is so effective.

Lawrence DE, Bennet PN: *Clinical Pharmacology*, ed 5. New York, Churchill Livingstone, 1981, pp 475–490.

A good account of human pharmacology of ethanol.

Lieber CS (ed): *Medical Disorders of Alcoholism.* Philadelphia, WB Saunders, 1982, vol 22, *Major Problems in Internal Medicine.*

A thorough coverage of alcohol-related diseases.

Moore MH, Gerstein DR (eds): *Alcohol and Public Policy: Beyond the Shadow of Prohibition.* Washington, DC, National Academy Press, 1981.

An important analysis of public-policy approaches to the control of alcoholic beverages. Points out how the normal drinker contributes to accidents and other adverse sequelae.

Ritchie JM: The aliphatic alcohols, in Goodman AG, Goodman LS, Rall TW, Murad F (eds): *The Pharmacological Basis of Therapeutics*, ed 7. New York, Macmillan, 1986, pp 372–386.

The standard account of ethanol pharmacology.

Vaillant GE: *The Natural History of Alcoholism: Causes, Patterns, and Paths to Recovery.* Cambridge, Mass, Harvard University Press, 1983.

A description of an influential prospective long-term study of the natural history of alcoholism.

West LJ (ed): *Alcoholism and Related Problems: Issues of the American Public.* The American Assembly, Columbia University. Englewood Cliffs, NJ, Prentice-Hall, 1984.

A provocative analysis of policy issues facing the American people.

Zook CJ, Moore FD: High cost users of medical care. *N Engl J Med* 1980;302: 996–1002.

An important paper documenting the impact of smoking and alcoholism on hospital-related health costs.

Primary Care of the Alcoholic Patient

Bean MH: Denial and the psychological complications of alcoholism, in Bean MH, Zinberg NE (eds): *Dynamic Approaches to the Understanding of Alcoholism.* New York, Free Press, 1981, pp 55–96.

A thorough, sensitive inquiry into the notion of denial. Although written by a psychiatrist, the illustrated case histories provide valuable insights for the general practicing physician.

Clark WD: Alcoholism: Blocks to diagnosis and treatment. *Am J Med* 1981; 71:275–286.

An internist's perspective on diagnosis and denial in office practice. A practical, clinical approach.

DiCicco L, Unterberger H, Mack JE: Confronting denial: An alcoholism intervention strategy. *Psychiatr Ann* 1978;8:596–606.

An excellent analysis of denial and caregiver's role in helping the developing alcoholic. Oriented toward the mental health professional.

Editors: Disulfiram (Antabuse). *Medical Letter.* New Rochelle, NY, 1980; 22(1):1.

A clinical review.

Emrick CD: A review of psychologically oriented treatment of alcoholism. II. The relative effectiveness of different treatment approaches and the effectiveness of treatment versus no treatment. *J Stud Alcohol* 1975;36:88–108.

A review of 384 studies of alcoholism treatment that concludes that there is no difference in the rate of achieving abstinence in untreated patients versus treated patients, but treated patients were more likely to improve.

Groves JE: Taking care of the hateful patient. *N Engl J Med* 1978;8:596–606.

The strategies outlined for approaching any difficult patient are particularly applicable to patients with alcoholism.

Hemmingsen R, Kramp P, Rafaelsen OS: Delirium tremens and related clinical states. Aetiology, pathophysiology and treatment. *Acta Psychiat Scand* 1979; 59:337–369.

Although many of the recommended therapies are not popular in this country, the authors' descriptions of the rationale for therapy are superb.

Kissin B: The role of physical dependence and brain damage in the protracted alcohol abstinence syndrome. *Adv Alcoholism* 1981;2(11):1–3.

An excellent review of the prolonged withdrawal syndrome with practical suggestions about management.

Kwentus J, Major LF: Disulfiram in the treatment of alcoholism. *J Stud Alcohol* 1979;40:428–446.

A comprehensive review of the mechanisms of action and disulfiram, its side effects and interactions with other drugs and alcohol.

Mayfield D, McLeod G, Hall P: The CAGE questionnaire: Validation of a new alcoholism screening instrument. *Am J Psychiatry* 1974;131:1121–1223.

The original study looking at the CAGE questionnaire applied to 366 patients admitted to a psychiatric service.

Naranjo CA, Sellers EM: Clinical assessment and pharmacotherapy of the alcohol withdrawal syndrome, in Galanter M (ed): *Recent Developments in Alcoholism*. New York, Plenum Press, 1986, vol 4.

An excellent summary and descriptive approach to the pharmacologic therapy of alcohol withdrawal.

Pendry ML, Maltzman IM, West LJ: Controlled drinking by alcoholics: new findings and a reevaluation of a major affirmative study. *Science* 1982;217: 169–175.

In this 10-year follow-up of 20 alcoholics previously reported to be controlled drinkers, only 1 patient continued to drink in a controlled fashion.

Sellers EM, Naranjo CA, Peachey JE: Drugs to decrease alcohol consumption. *N Engl J Med* 1981;305:1255–1261.

Useful discussion of the clinical pharmacology of disulfiram.

Sellers EM, Kalant H: Alcohol intoxication and withdrawal. *N Engl J Med* 1976; 294:757–762.

Good section on intoxication; does not address outpatient management explicitly.

Skinner HA, Holt S, Israel Y: Early identification of alcohol abuse. 1. Critical issues and psychosocial indicators for a composite index. *Can Med Assoc J* 1981;124:1141–1150. 2. Clinical and laboratory indicators. *Can Med Assoc J* 1981;124:1279–1294.

This two-part article is an excellent, thorough review of the psychosocial problems, physical complaints, and laboratory abnormalities which may be associated with early alcoholism.

Skinner HA, Holt S, Schuler R, Israel Y: Identification of alcohol abuse using laboratory tests and a history of trauma. *Ann Intern Med* 1984;101:847–857.

A trauma scale derived from five questions about trauma is more sensitive than laboratory work in the identification of alcoholism.

Vaillant GE: *The Natural History of Alcoholism: Causes, Patterns, and Paths to Recovery.* Cambridge, Mass, Harvard University Press, 1983.

A statistical analysis of data from different populations examining predisposing factors in the development of alcoholism and the natural history of the disease.

Resources in the Community and Workplace

Baekeland F: Evaluation of treatment methods in chronic alcoholism, in Kissin B, Begleiter H (eds): *The Biology of Alcoholism*. New York, Plenum Press, 1977, vol 5, *Treatment and Rehabilitation of the Chronic Alcoholic*, pp 385–440.

A review of available literature on AA with particular attention to characteristics of AA members and the effectiveness of AA.

Dean MH: Alcoholics Anonymous. *Psychiatr Ann* 1975;5(2):7–61.

Interesting five-part series on AA, including psychodynamic formulation and critique of AA. The first sections are a good introduction to how AA works.

Curlee J: How a therapist can use Alcoholics Anonymous. *Ann NY Acad Sci* 1974;233:137–143.

A description of how AA provides role models and a stable social network that can be useful to the alcoholic and therapist in confronting denial.

Erfurt JC, Foote A: *Occupational Employee Assistance Programs for Substance Abuse and Mental Health Problems*. Ann Arbor, Worker Health Program, Institute of Labor and Industrial Relations, University of Michigan and Wayne State University, 1977.

This monograph develops a model for employee-assistance programs, emphasizing the distinction between functions performed internally in the company and those referred to outside contractors or providers.

Kurtz NR, Googins B, Howard WC: Measuring the success of occupational alcohol programs. *J Stud Alcohol* 1984;45:33–45.

A review of evaluation research on occupational alcoholism programs. The article includes speculation on why the literature is so weak and recommendations for future studies.

Shain M, Groeneveld J: *Employee-assistance Programs*. Lexington, Mass, Lexington Books, 1980.

A comprehensive and critical analysis of the philosophy, theory, and practice of employee-assistance programs.

Vaillant GH: Dangers of psychotherapy in the treatment of alcoholism, in Bean MH, Zinberg NE (eds): *Dynamic Approaches to the Understanding and Treatment of Alcoholism*. New York, Free Press, 1981, pp 55–96.

Starting with the premise that alcoholism is a primary disease, the author describes an outpatient treatment program based on the concepts, but not the structure of AA. A compelling case history illustrates his point of view.

Walsh DC: Employee assistance programs. *Millbank Mem Fund Q/Health Soc* 1982;60:492–517.

A review and analysis of the historical and philosophical underpinnings of the EAP movement.

Wrich JT: *Guidelines for Developing an Employee Assistance Program*. New York, American Management Assoc, 1982.

A concise handbook, this monograph describes procedures for implementation of an EAP program, considerations of costs and benefits and some issues associated with evaluation.

Pathophysiology and Medical Complications

Brechot C, et al: Evidence that hepatitis B virus has a role in liver cell carcinoma in alcoholic liver disease. *N Engl J Med* 1982;306:1384–1387.

This study demonstrates a higher rate of HBV integrated into liver cells in alcoholics with HCC compared to those without HCC.

Breeden JH: Alcohol, alcoholism, and cancer. *Med Clin North Am* 1984;68: 163–177.

A very good and comprehensive review of the subject. It includes mechanisms of carcinogenesis, sites affected, and problems associated with treating the alcoholic cancer patient. Extensive bibliography.

Burbige EJ, Lewis DR Jr, Halstead CH: Alcohol and the gastrointestinal tract. *Med Clin North Am* 1984;68(1):77–89.

Thorough review of the literature. Alcohol's effects on the esophagus, stomach, and small intestine are reviewed.

Cahill GF Jr: Nephrology Forum. Ketosis. *Kidney Int* 1982;20:416–425.

A detailed physiologic exposition of the processes responsible for ketosis; a patient with diabetes suffering from starvation and alcohol abuse is the focus of discussion.

Clarren SK, Smith DW: The fetal alcohol syndrome. *N Engl J Med* 1978;298: 1063–1067.

The clinical features of the syndrome are described. Information on the impact and the epidemiology of the fetal alcohol syndrome may be found in the referenced articles.

Dirks JH: Nephrology Forum. The kidney and magnesium regulation. *Kidney Int* 1983;23:771–777.

A concise summary of normal and abnormal renal magnesium metabolism including a brief discussion of the clinical causes of hypomagnesemia.

Editorial: Alcoholic brain damage. *Lancet* 1981;1:477–478.

A useful, historical perspective about the trend toward a more unitary view of clinical syndromes resulting from alcohol's effect on the brain.

Geokas MC: Ethanol and the pancreas. *Med Clin North Am* 1984;68(1):57–75.

Highly readable, concise overview of pathophysiologic and clinical aspects of acute and chronic alcoholic pancreatitis.

Green HR: Alcohol, nutrition, and malabsorption. *Clin Gastroenterol* 1983; 12(2):563–575.

Excellent summary of the mechanisms of malabsorption in the chronic alcoholic. The direct and indirect effects of alcohol on small intestinal morphology and function and their impact on malnutrition are covered.

Harrington JT, Cohen JJ, Kassirer JP: Mixed acid–base disturbances, in Cohen JJ, Kassirer JP (ed): *Acid–Base*. Boston, Little, Brown, and Company, 1982.

An analytic review of all the mixed acid–base disorders, including those seen in alcoholics.

Herbert V (ed): Hematologic complications of alcoholism. *Semin Hematol* 1980; 17:83–176.

This scholarly symposium details all the hematologic disorders associated with alcohol.

Lieber CS, Leo MA: Alcohol and the liver, in Lieber CS (ed): *Medical Disorders of Alcoholism: Pathogenesis and Treatment*. Philadelphia, WB Saunders, 1982, pp 259–312.

A good, comprehensive review with emphasis on pathophysiology.

Lishman WA: Cerebral disorder in alcoholism: Syndromes of impairment. *Brain* 1981;104:1–20.

An excellent review of the Wernicke-Korsakoff syndrome, alcoholic dementia, and cerebral atrophy.

McCoy GD, Wynder EL: Etiological and preventive implications in alcohol carcinogenesis. *Cancer Res* 1979;29:2844–2850.

A discussion of the epidemiology and possible mechanisms whereby alcohol may be related to carcinogenesis.

Morgan MY: Alcohol and nutrition. *Br Med Bull* 1982;38:21–29.

A comprehensive treatment of the nutritional problems of alcoholism, emphasizing pathophysiology.

Nakada T, Knight RT: Alcohol and the central nervous system. *Med Clin North Am* 1984;68:121–131.

An excellent view of the neurologic complications, with 35 references.

Popper S: Hepatorenal syndrome, in Epstein M (ed): *The Kidney in Liver Disease*. New York, Elsevier, 1983.

A current synthesis of the basic and clinical aspects of this deadly disease.

Rankin JGD, Orreggo-Matte H, Deschenes J, et al: Alcoholic liver disease: The problem of diagnosis. *Alcoholism Clin Exp Res* 1978;2:327–338.

Uses 100 patients with histologic diagnosis to demonstrate the poor correlation between clinical and laboratory data and histologic diagnosis and poor correlation of history and functional status and prognosis.

Regan TJ, Haider B: Ethanol abuse and heart disease. *Circulation* 1981;64(III): 14–19.

This is a well-referenced clinical summary of the diverse manifestations of alcohol heart disease.

Reuler JB, Girard DE, Cooney TG: Wernicke's encephalopathy. *N Engl J Med*, 1985;312:1035–1039.

An up-to-date review of Wernicke's encephalopathy with an excellent discussion about prevention.

Ritz E: Nephrology Forum. Acute hypophosphatemia. *Kidney Int*, 1981;22: 89–94.

A review of the pathophysiology of phosphate depletion and its myriad manifestations.

Schenker S: Alcoholic liver disease: Evaluation of natural history and prognostic factors. *Hepatology* 1984;4:36S–43S.

A good review of major natural history studies and discussion of roles of prognostic factors.

Schmidt W, Popham RE: The role of drinking and smoking in mortality from cancer and other causes in male alcoholics. *Cancer* 1981;47:1031–1041.

This study examined mortality in 9,889 males and compared it with deaths expected from different causes; it then looked for excess deaths compared with nonalcoholic smokers.

Tuyns AJ, Pequinot G: Greater risk of ascitic cirrhosis in females in relation to alcohol consumption. *Int J Epidemiol* 1984;13:53–57.

A case-control study to assess relative risk for cirrhosis in males and females for various levels of alcohol consumption: Women are at increased risk at lower levels of alcohol consumption.

Valencia-Parparcen J: Alcoholic gastritis. *Clin Gastroenterol* 1981;10(2):389–399.

Comprehensive review of relationship between alcohol and acute and chronic gastritis: pathogenesis, diagnosis, symptomatology, and treatment.

Van Thiel DH, Gavaler JS, Sanghvi A: Recovery of sexual function in abstinent alcoholic men. *Gastroenterology* 1982;84:677–682.

The prognosis for alcohol-induced impotence is favorable.

Victor M: Neurologic aspects of alcoholism, in Feldman RG (ed): *Neurology: The Physician's Guide*. New York, Thieme-Stratton Inc. 1984, pp 178–190.

This chapter is a clinician's guide to the neurologic complications of alcoholism, with particular emphasis on problems encountered in inner city hospitals.

Williams RR, Horm JW: Association of cancer sites with tobacco and alcohol consumption and socioeconomic status of patients: Interview study from the Third National Cancer Survey. *J Natl Cancer Inst* 1977;58:525–547.

A correlation of interview data on the above variables with cancer at various sites.

Alcohol and Special Populations

Atkinson RM, Lofoed LL: Alcohol and drug abuse in old age, in Cassal C, Walsh JR (eds): *Geriatric Medicine*. New York, Springer-Verlag, 1984, vol 2, *Fundamentals of Geriatric Care*, pp 219–235.

An excellent, thorough review of alcohol abuse in the elderly, placing it in the context of patterns of drug abuse. Risk factors, diagnosis, prevalence, and clinical presentations are well covered.

Bean M: Identifying and managing alcohol problems in adolescents. *Psychosomatics* 1982;23(4):389–396.

In this brief, clinical article, Bean differentiates normal experimentation, problem drinking, and alcoholism in adolescents and describes a clinical approach to the teenage problem drinker.

Beckman LJ, Amaro H: Patterns of women's use of alcohol treatment agencies, in Wilsnack SC, Beck LJ (eds): *Alcohol Problems in Women*. New York, The Guilford Press, 1983.

Discusses barriers that impede female problem drinkers from both entering into and continuing in treatment.

Black C: *It Will Never Happen to Me*. Denver, Medical Administration Company, 1982.

This book has poignant chapters describing the problems of children of alcoholics.

Craddock SG, Brady RM, Hubbard RL: *Drug Use Before and During Drug Abuse Treatment*: 1979–1981, TOPS admission cohorts. DHHS Publication No (ADM) 85-1387, 1985;13–30.

This first report on a large-scale, longitudinal study examines the profile of drug users, their patterns of drug use, and outcome of treatment based on type of therapeutic program.

Department of Health and Human Services: *Fourth Special Report to the US Congress on Alcohol and Health*. 1981:81–1080.

The report covers patterns of drinking, drinking problems, medical and social consequences of alcohol abuse, prevention, and treatment.

Dykens JW, Bayog RD: The treatment of drug addiction, in Wolman BB (ed): *The Therapist's Handbook*. New York, Van Nostrand Rheinhold, 1983, pp 483–505.

Reviews the current literature including epidemiology, the biopsychosocial determinants, specific treatment issues, strategies, and approaches to commonly used addicting drugs. Instruction and a ready reference on clinical matters during various stages of treatment.

Gerbino PP: Complications of alcohol use combined with drug therapy in the elderly. *J Am Geriatr Soc* 1982;30(suppl):S88–S93.

This brief review summarizes the pharmacology of alcohol and presents potentially significant or dangerous drug–alcohol interactions most commonly encountered in an elderly population.

Gomberg ESL: Alcohol use and alcohol problems among the elderly, in *Alcohol and Health, Special Population Issues*, Monograph No 4. Rockville, Md, National Institute on Alcohol Abuse and Alcoholism, 1982:263–290.

Epidemiology and natural history of elderly drinkers are discussed in this chapter highlighting the problems of identifying and following the clinical and social course of older drinkers.

Grant I, Adams K, Reed R: Aging, abstinence and medical risk factors in the prediction of neuropsychological deficit among long-term alcoholics. *Arch Gen Psychiatry* 1984;41:710–718.

This study attempts to identify the contributions of remote and recent abstinence and the interaction of aging on neuropsychologic testing of long-term alcoholics. A thoughtful discussion of the premature aging hypothesis is included.

Hamilton G, Volpe J: How women recover: Experience and research observations. *Alcohol Health Res World* 1982/3;7:28–39.

An article based on a conference of representatives of 40 of the 45 women's treatment programs funded during the preceding 11 years by the National Institute on Alcohol Abuse and Alcoholism plus a review of the literature related to women's treatment issues raised by conference participants.

Hartford JT, Samorajski T (eds): *Alcoholism in the Elderly.* New York, Raven Press, 1984.

This excellent text focuses on the physiologic rather than the social aspects of the problem. Animal alcohol research is discussed, as are the physiologic and cognitive changes associated with aging and alcohol.

Hill SY: Biological consequences of alcoholism and alcohol-related problems among women, in *Alcohol and Health, Special Population Issues*, Monograph No 4. Rockville, Md, National Institute on Alcohol Abuse and Alcoholism, 1982:43–76.

Compares the prevalence of biomedical consequences of alcohol abuse in men and women.

Jackson JK: The adjustment of the family to the crisis of alcoholism. *Q J Stud Alcohol* 1954;15:562–586.

A paper of historical interest that discusses how families adjust to an alcoholic member as seen from the perspective of wives of alcoholics.

Johnson VE: *I'll Quit Tomorrow: A Practical Guide to Alcoholism*, rev ed. San Francisco, Harper & Row, 1980.

A classic. Must reading for all who wish to understand alcoholism as seen through the eyes of a recovered alcoholic.

Mayer J, Filstead W: The adolescent alcohol involvement scale. *J Stud Alcohol* 1979;40:291–300.

The adolescent alcohol involvement scale is an instrument designed to obtain a deeper history of an adolescent's drinking patterns and problems than a conventional review of systems questions, such as "How much do you drink?" which can cause a patient to react defensively. It can be used in the office as a springboard to discussion after the teenager completes the questionnaire and the physician reviews it with him.

Meyer RE: *Guide to Drug Rehabilitation, A Public Health Response.* Boston, Beacon Press, 1972.

Reviews existing major treatment modalities for drug rehabilitation. It is practical, comprehensive, and has an excellent overview of therapeutic responses in treating specific drug problems.

Mishara BL, Kastenbaum R: *Alcohol and Old Age*. New York, Grune & Stratton, 1980, pp 127–162.

This text is a well-balanced review of problem drinking among the elderly and the beneficial effects of alcohol use in old age. Included are discussions on the physiologic effect of alcohol, the extent of its use in this population, and problems associated with such use. Treatment approaches are well reviewed.

Morse RM, Martin MA, Swenson WM, Niven RG: Prognosis of physicians treated for alcoholism and drug dependence. *JAMA* 1984;251:743–746.

The prognosis for physicians in this Mayo Clinic-treated population was more favorable than for general patients. Eighty-three percent of physicians and 62% of the general group had favorable outcomes. Close monitoring accounted, in part, for the better prognosis of physicians.

Rachal JV, Maisto SA, Guess LL, Hubbard RL: Alcohol use among adolescents, in *Alcohol Consumption and Related Problems*. Alcohol and Health Monograph No 1. Rockville, Md, National Institute of Alcohol Abuse and Alcoholism, 1981.

These social scientists have carried out some of the largest and most methodologically satisfactory studies of alcohol use and difficulties adolescents face. Statistical, rather than clinical, their findings nevertheless suggest that clinicians ought to be seeing more adolescents with alcohol problems.

Sandmaier M: *The Invisible Alcoholics: Women and Alcohol in America*. New York, McGraw-Hill, 1980.

A comprehensive overview of alcoholism among American women based on an extensive literature review and interviews with alcoholism specialists and 50 recovered alcoholics from various backgrounds.

Schuckit MA: *Drug and Alcohol Abuse*. New York, Plenum Press, 1984.

An excellent clinical reference on learning the classes of drugs of abuse, understanding their psychopharmacology, management of emergencies, and rehabilitation.

Schuckit MA, Morrisey ER: Alcoholism in women: Some clinical and social perspectives with an emphasis on possible subtypes, in Greenblatt M, Schuckit MA (eds): *Alcoholism Problems in Women and Children*. New York, Grune & Stratton, 1976, pp 5–36.

A selective literature review of alcoholism in women, with an emphasis on comparisons between male and female alcoholics.

Spickard A Jr, Billings FT: Alcoholism in a medical school faculty. *N Engl J Med* 1981;305:1646–1648.

The authors report experiences with alcoholic faculty members in a medical school and suggest approaches for improving care for colleagues.

Spickard A, Thompson BR: *Dying for a Drink—What You Should Know about Alcoholism*. Waco, Tex, Word Publishers, Inc., 1985, pp 102–136.

This book describes the authors' experiences in caring for alcoholics and their families, emphasizing early identification, intervention, and recovery.

Steinglass P: Experimenting with family treatment approaches to alcoholism, 1950–1975: A review. *Fam Process* 1976;15:97–123.

A comprehensive but dated review of various family treatment approaches to alcoholism.

Stitzer ML, Bigelow GE, McCaul ME: *Behavior Therapy in Drug Abuse Treatment: Review and Evaluation*. DHHS Publication No ADM 85-1401, 1985: 31–50.

This article describes a behavioral model of drug abuse and suggests four behavioral therapy strategies with applications in treatment.

Talbott GD, Martin CA: Relapse and recovery: Special issues for chemically dependent physicians. *J Med Assoc Ga* 1984;73:763–769.

A review of the special circumstances most frequently observed as factors contributing to relapse after treatment for chemical dependency.

Thoreson RW: The professor at risk: Alcohol abuse in academe, in Thoreson RW, Hosokawa EP (eds): *Employee Assistance Programs in Higher Education*. Springfield, Ill, Charles C Thomas, 1984, pp 123–143.

This book is an extensive overview of the development and adaptation of employee-assistance programming in higher education. The book focuses on means of enhancing the academic environment for faculty and staff.

Wegscheider S: *Another Chance*. Palo Alto, Science and Behavior Books, Inc, 1981.

An excellent book that discusses the dynamics of the alcoholic family in an easily readable fashion.

Legal Issues in the Treatment of Alcoholism

Beauchamp T, Childress J: *Principles of Biomedical Ethics*. New York, Oxford University Press, 1983.

A classic text on the nature and principles of biomedical ethics. The authors discuss the principles of autonomy, nonmalfeasance, justice, and confidentiality.

Childress J: *Who Should Decide? Paternalism in Health Care*. New York, Oxford University Press, 1982.

A comprehensive analysis of paternalism in the health care system focusing on definitions and implications. Broad ethical principles, such as autonomy and beneficence, are discussed in addition to specific case–study material.

Katz J: *The Silent World of Doctor and Patient.* New York, Free Press, 1984.

An insightful text focusing on informed consent, autonomy, and the nature of the doctor–patient relationship. The text is theoretical as well as practical.

US Department of Transportation. *Fatal Accident Reporting System, 1984.* DOT HS 806 919, 1986.

This volume reports on the characteristics of fatal crashes in the United States, including type of vehicle, roadway, use of seatbelt, and presence of alcohol. Data include state and national summaries.

Index

MIX
Papier aus verantwortungsvollen Quellen
Paper from responsible sources
FSC® C105338
www.fsc.org

If you have any concerns about our products,
you can contact us on
ProductSafety@springernature.com

In case Publisher is established outside the EU,
the EU authorized representative is:
Springer Nature Customer Service Center GmbH
Europaplatz 3, 69115 Heidelberg, Germany

Printed by Libri Plureos GmbH
in Hamburg, Germany